COMPLEX REGIONA

PATIENTS' PERSPECTIVE OF LIVING IN CHRONIC PAIN

Volume 1

By

Alaa Abd-Elsayed M.D., MPH, FASA and Eric M. Phillips

To: DR S,   2-11-20

Thank-you for
being a great Doctor
and for helping my Pain.

Best Wishes!

Eric

First edition, 2020

Volume 1

ISBN: 9781657371149

Other books published by authors:

Alaa Abd-Elsayed

- Chronic Pain: The Patient and Family Journey
- If the Savior is not Safe, How Can He Save?
- Pain: A Review Guide
- Infusion Therapy for Pain, Headache and Related Conditions

Dedication

To my parents, my wife and my two beautiful kids Maro and George.

To all CRPS patients.

Alaa Abd-Elsayed

Dedication

To my loving parents, Janet and my late father Leonard (Lenny) Phillips for all their love, and support.

To my beautiful and supportive wife Mercedes, her three children and her grandson.

To my mentor, teacher and greatest friend the late Doctor Hooshang Hooshmand.

To all RSD-CRPS patients worldwide.

Eric M. Phillips

TABLE OF CONTENTS

Preface

First, I would like to thank all patients who were willing to share their stories in this book. I have been a pain physician for several years and Complex Regional Pain Syndrome (CRPS) has been one of the conditions that I specialize in. I have seen cases very early in the disease and cases very late in the disease, I have seen patients who have been around for years, misdiagnosed or not diagnosed at all, I have seen patients who, when treated early, recover completely and patients when not treated appropriately lose function, lose a limb and may commit suicide.

I had the pleasure of knowing my friend Eric Phillips through a clinical trial I was involved in for treating CRPS, we provided advice for some patients and our friendship continued since then.

We decided to author and edit this book to increase the awareness of the public and medical providers about CRPS as a condition where the pain can kill, leads to death and serious disability. Our goal is to share it with health care providers, so they take the condition seriously and treat it aggressively. We want the professionals to know that the pain is real and those patients are not seeking drugs, but they are looking for a cure for their pain.

We also want the public to learn about the disease to support patients who could be their friends, their family or their beloved ones. THE PAIN IS REAL AND SEVERE.

I hope this book will provide good information to all and will increase awareness about the disease.

Alaa Abd-Elsayed, MD, MPH, FASA

Preface

I would like to especially thank all the CRPS patients for taking the time to write and share their stories. It is generous of all of you to share your journey of living with this painful disease in this book. Your willingness to share your story will provide great help and support to others who are suffering from CRPS.

I have been working in the CRPS community for over 31-years to help advocate for other CRPS patients. As, being a sufferer of CRPS myself for over 34-years, I understand the struggles and pain that CRPS patients endure. The biggest downfall for most patients is the lack of understanding of CRPS by the medical community.

I have been fortunate to know and work with my friend Doctor Alaa Abd-Elsayed over the years. It has been a great honor for me to work on this book with Doctor Al and all the patients that were so gracious enough to submit their stories.

We both felt that writing a book that shared patient's personal stories would help spread the desperately needed awareness, help educate the public and the medical community that CRPS is a "real" disease.

I hope this book will be helpful and provide reassurance to other CRPS patients that they are not alone; with their daily battle of dealing with the chronic pain of CRPS. Moreover, I also hope this book will help the medical community worldwide to understand how patients live and cope with this unrelenting painful disease.

Eric M. Phillips

COMPLEX REGIONAL PAIN SYNDROME (CRPS)
By: Alaa Abd-Elsayed, MD, MPH, FASA

Complex regional pain syndrome (CRPS), also called reflex sympathetic dystrophy syndrome (RSD) is a syndrome characterized by chronic pain due to a high level of nerve impulses sent to the affected limb.

The syndrome can affect children and has been reported in women more than men.

Classically CRPS is classified into two types:
Type 1: CRPS following a trivial injury as a fracture or sprain.
Type 2: CRPS following a major injury as a trauma or surgery causing a serious nerve injury.

The distinction between both types can sometimes be difficult and several entities have been advocating for removing this classification.

Mechanism of CRPS
Focal small-fiber axonal degeneration and alteration of the cutaneous innervation by small-diameter fibers can play a role in the development of CRPS. The condition is multifactorial with a genetic predisposition. It also involves peripheral sensitization at the site of injury and central sensitization, which makes the condition very severe and leads to the exaggerated pain on touch, pressure and any other mild stimuli. In CRPS there is an alteration in the sympathetic nervous system. Psychological factors as anxiety can make the condition worse and it is commonly present in patients with CRPS due to the seriousness of the condition and its impact on the patient and family.

Symptoms
Based on the Budapest Criteria, for a diagnosis of CRPS, a patient must have at least one symptom in three of the following four categories:

Sensory: hyperesthesia (an abnormal increase in sensitivity) and/or allodynia (pain caused by usually non-painful stimuli).

Vasomotor: skin color changes or temperature and/or skin color changes between the limbs.

Sudomotor/edema: edema (swelling) and/or sweating changes and/or sweating differences between the limbs.

Motor/trophic: decreased range of motion and/or motor dysfunction (weakness, tremor, muscular spasm (dystonia)) and/or trophic changes (changes to the hair and/or nail and/or skin on the limb).

Signs
At the time of clinical examination, at least, one sign must be present in two or more of the following categories:

Sensory: hyperalgesia (to pinprick) and/or allodynia (to light touch and/or deep somatic (physical) pressure and/or joint movement).

Vasomotor: temperature differences between the limbs and/or skin color changes and/or skin color changes between the limbs.

Sudomotor/edema: edema and/or sweating changes and/or sweating differences between the limbs.

Motor/trophic: decreased range of motion and/or motor dysfunction (i.e., weakness, tremor, or muscle spasm) and/or trophic changes (hair and/or nail and/or skin changes).

In addition, it is important that no other diagnosis can explain the signs and symptoms.

It is very important to provide the appropriate treatment and early in the disease to avoid the development of adverse outcomes. Management can be established using the following modalities.

Non-pharmacological management
Physical therapy, occupational therapy, heat and cold therapy, relaxation techniques, pain psychology and more should be tried first.

Medications
- Non-steroidal anti-inflammatory drugs (NSAIDs).
- Anticonvulsants, such as gabapentin.
- Topical creams and patches.
- Corticosteroids.
- Bisphosphonates.
- Opioids after performing a risk assessment and discussing risks and benefits.
- N-methyl-D-aspartate (NMDA) receptor antagonists.

Interventions
Sympathetic nerve blocks.
Spinal cord stimulation.
Intrathecal drug delivery.
Surgical sympathectomy.

Experimental therapies
- Intravenous immunoglobulin.
- Capsaicin.
- Amputation.

Complications
- Chest pain.
- Problems with thinking and memory.
- Lethargy, fatigue, and weakness.

- Rapid pulse and heart palpitations.
- Breathing problems.
- Fluid retention.
- Muscle weakness and bone loss.
- Rashes, mottling and skin discoloration.
- Urological problems such as difficulty urinating or incontinence.
- Gastrointestinal problems, including nausea, vomiting, diarrhea, and Irritable bowel syndrome (IBS).
- Gastroesophageal reflux.
- Low cortisol levels and hypothyroidism.
- Loss of function in the affected limb due to lack of use, atrophy, contractures and severe pain.

References

- Goh EL, Chidambaram S, Ma D. Complex regional pain syndrome: a recent update. Burns Trauma. 2017 Jan 19; 5:2.
- Bruehl S, Chung OY. Psychological and behavioral aspects of complex regional pain syndrome management. Clin J Pain. 2006 Jun;22(5):430-7.
- Maihöfner C, Birklein F. [Complex regional pain syndromes: new aspects on pathophysiology and therapy]. Fortschr Neurol Psychiatr. 2007 Jun;75(6):331-42.
- Wasner G, Schattschneider J, Binder A, Baron R. Complex regional pain syndrome--diagnostic, mechanisms, CNS involvement and therapy. Spinal Cord. 2003 Feb;41(2):61-75.
- Bruehl S. An update on the pathophysiology of complex regional pain syndrome. Anesthesiology. 2010 Sep;113(3):713-25.

MY LIFE WITH ALGODYSTROPHY
By: Cécile Moreau

On October 02, 2012, I was a victim of a car accident while going to work. I was stopped at a red light when a car hit me in the back, causing material and physical damage. Initially, the lesions were as follows:

- ➢ sprained with both hands,
- ➢ cervical sprain,
- ➢ moving vertebrae and pelvis,
- ➢ internal contusions on the belly.

Given my professional situation (director of a private higher education institution and professor of law / economics / tourism marketing), I did not stop working, but only in TA with the obligation of care, so I could continue to work.

After three weeks, the lesions eased, except on my right hand. My doctor gave me a splint for three extra weeks, but still no evolution. I then consulted a hand specialist who ordered an ultrasound, which showed hyperthermia of the hand with edema. He even infiltrated, which aggravated my condition. I stayed for 10-months with intense pain without anyone making a diagnosis. In August of 2013, I was feeling exhausted physically and morally so, I decided to make an appointment at the Georges Pompidou European Hospital in Paris to see a hand trauma specialist. This doctor diagnosed me with a cold-phase dystrophy. The only problem is that it was too late to undertake some care. The doctor explained to me the phases of the dystrophy. He concluded that there could be a small chance of me recovering the functionality of my hand. You must know that I am right-handed and that the consequences have been disastrous.

My health has deteriorated over the years. Today, I still suffer from a cold-phase dystrophy of the dominant right hand and the shoulder with right hemithorax pain radiating to the lower back. I had various analgesic treatments that had little effect and I had to stop because of drug poisoning.

I have gone to the Functional Rehabilitation Center twice. This is where I worked with a physiotherapist, occupational therapy, balneotherapy, light fitness, and psychological follow-up, in the hopes of an upgrade. Unfortunately, we have not found sufficient positive evolution related notably to the pain limiting daily gestures. I do physiotherapy three to four times a week and wear a brace day and night. In September of 2015, I was no longer able to withstand the pain of the algodystrophy (AGD) (which is the French term for complex regional pain syndrome (CRPS), I decided to have a neurostimulator medullary. I had to adhere to the following daily instructions, namely not to:

- ➢ Raise your arms
- ➢ Driving (I have to travel 6 kms to physio)
- ➢ To lean
- ➢ To lower myself
- ➢ Twisting with the upper body
- ➢ Play sports...

In short, anything that can have an impact on my healing is forbidden.

But my career with Miss A does not stop there!... In September 2016, new intervention to reposition my electrode that had migrated. Fifteen days after the operation, I began to feel terrible pain all over my body. I ended up being hospitalized in December 2016. The doctors concluded that I was rejecting my device. My neurosurgeon does not think that my neurostimulator is at risk. I had to wait for a new bone scan in July 2018 to confirm what my GP was suspecting: namely a migration of the dystrophy on my left foot.

The problem is that in France, doctors do not want to recognize the migration of AGD and tell us that " it's in our head." I refuse to believe and think. Fortunately, my neurosurgeon is more open-minded and understood my problem.

On March 28, 2019, he put me another electrode positioned at T9, and T11 to relieve my pain.

To date, after six years with the algodystrophy, I continue the fight. She is always present, more than ever ... I do physio three times a week, hypnosis, reiki, relaxation, and tests alternative medicine. I do not despair of getting out one day, but I no longer have any illusions about my functional recovery. I learn every day to live with my disability. But I lost a lot in the battle: my job; my social life, my friends, some of my family members, and the life of a couple is difficult.

EVOLUTION HEALTH CONDITION FOLLOWING CAR ACCIDENT OF 02 OCTOBER 2012- SUMMARY DATED 03 SEPTEMBER 2018

On October 2, 2012, I was the victim of an AVP, recognized as an accident by the Social Security. I was stopped at a red light when a car hit me from behind, about 70 kms.

Oct 2, 2012:
Exams performed: hand radio and cervico-dorso-lumbar radio.
Conclusions: *"Cervical sprain C4,C5 minimal left C2,C3 narrowing; moderate disc disease L1,L2 minimal right pelvis rocker higher than the left of 3 mm, left peri- cotyloid calcification in favor of insertion tendinopathy; moderate nipping of L4,L5 and L5,S1 discs rather on the right side"*, belly contusions; sprains e to x both hands.

A few weeks later, recovery except at the level of the right hand, very painful, red, shiny and with edema. Difficulties to mobilize it.

2013

Jan / Feb 2013: Persistent pain right hand

Exams performed: ultrasound (11.01.2013); MRI (15.02 2013)
Conclusions: RAS for both exams.

From Feb 2013 to   July 2013: Consultations with Doctor R, orthopedic surgeon specialized in the hand at Clinique du Parc in Lyon. He does not understand why the pain persists despite the use of various treatments as well as analgesic and anti-inflammatory treatments. Exams performed: ultrasound of the hand (26.02.2013); infiltration (10.05.2013); radio (04.06.13); scintigraphy (24.07.2013); MSD EMG (25.07.2013)

Conclusions: Echo: *"arthro -synovite trapezo -métacarpienne   with minimal effusion (pain at the passage of the probe) and power Doppler hypervascularisation; hyperthermia at the level of the enthesis of the short flexor tendon of the right thumb on the lateral sesamoid with clear pain at the passage of the probe."* Infiltration: xylocaine and diprstene Radio: no damage to the scaphoid scintigraphy: RAS EMG: RAS

Despite the use of analgesics, anti-inflammatories, physiotherapy (massage and cryotherapy) and infiltration, the pain persists and worsens. More and more difficulties in using my hand, especially after infiltration.

August   12,   2013: Consultation in a hand trauma department Hospital Georges Pompidou Paris.
Conclusion: *After clinical examination and different shots, diagnosis of algo-neuro dystrophy cold phase of MSD with sequelae.*

Sept 17, 2013: Consultation with Doctor C, a sports doctor.
Conclusion: *Temperature decreased by one to two degrees between the right and left hand. Stiffness of all fingers right hand; a little sensation of increased perspiration.*

Confirmation of cold-phase dysrhythmias dystrophy.

Setting up a mild physiotherapist more analgesic. But persisting pains that now to go up in the wrist, elbow, and shoulder.

2014

Jan 13, 2014: Consultation with Doctor R, a neurologist.
Conclusion: *Confirmation of algoneurodystrophie; implementation of Lyrica, physio and TENS. Pain that still does not give way.*

Feb 2014: Supported by Doctor DS, a psychiatrist at Irigny. Follow-up already in progress to date once a month.
Treatment: One deroxat in the evening, deleted in 2017 because useless.

March 26, 2014: Consultation with Doctor P, a rheumatologist.
Conclusion: " *Today's examination shows a cold right hand with dry skin, a spontaneous position in flexion of the fingers with a clear increase in pain during the extension of all the fingers. The mobilization of the p o in is painful but does not seem limited. These arguments are in favor of a cold phase dysphasy dystrophy.*" Proposal for a spa treatment (not performed) and taken in CAD (refusal). Wearing a resting splint at night and a day splint. Continuation of TENS and Lyrica. Still no positive evolution.

June/July 2014: Complete hospitalization at the Marseille Valmante Functional Rehabilitation Center. Set up of occupational therapy, physiotherapy, balneotherapy and fitness sessions "athletic." At the exit small improvement but nothing blatant.

July 1, 2014: Cervical spine CT for an indication of frequent headaches and vertigo.
Conclusions: " *C5, C6 disc disease with narrowing of the inter-somatic interline and posterior medial posterior protrusion effacing the anterior epidural space. Disc disease C6, C7 with medial posterior protrusion more discrete.*"

Nov 2014: AIT (suspicion of stroke) found by Doctor R with HTA. Establishment of treatment with Kardegic 75mg and Icaz 5mg.

The year continues, but always with my right arm and upper back pain resistant to any type of therapy.

2015

Many drug intolerances appear. Discontinuation of treatments except for doliprane. The pains are more and more poorly supported and evolve in the back. It has been discussed the possibility of setting up a spinal neurostimulator if rehabilitation still does not give anything.

Jul / Aug 2015: Hospitalization at CRF Valmante but no efficacy.
Sept 2015: Placement of the medullary neurostimulator by Doctor B at Clinique Charcot. Electrode positioned in C7 and Medtronic case in the right iliac fossa. Reduction of pain without finding the functionality of the hand.

2016
Despite the placement of the neurostimulator, which significantly improved pain and physiotherapy sessions three to four times a week, no functional recovery. So, I asked to be hospitalized at CRF Valmante. In July 2016, Doctor L.G., refuses to take me back. She explains this by the fact that " *it's algoneurodystrophie is old at the moment and the sequelae a permanent priority, at least at the functional level.*" In parallel, the neurostimulator becomes less effective.

Sept 2016: Repositioning of the electrode that has migrated.

Oct 2016: Very sharp pains appear at the level of the lower back and extend progressively at the level of the legs then feet.

Dec 2016: Hospitalization of 10-days in the rheumatology department of the St. Joseph-St. Luc Hospital in Lyon because the pains in the whole body are unbearable. Laroxyl + cortisone infusions and oral pain relief.
Review realized: MRI cervical spine (07.12.2016)
Conclusion: *"Herniated disc added and without distal radicular conflict at C4, C5, C6, and C7."* During this hospitalization, the doctors wonder if my electrode would not be badly positioned and thus at the origin of these new pains. Doctor B thinks no. Stopping the drugs because of cortisone intolerance and Laroxyl.

2017

Jan 25, 2017: Urgent consultation (because I had gone to see my family) with Doctor L, neurosurgeon hospital Beauregard Marseille following a new crisis of violent back pain, legs, and feet.
Conclusion: *"The repositioning of the right-side electrode should be considered at the same level. "*

Feb 7, 2017: Consultation with Doctor B, a neurosurgeon. After seeing the MRI in December 2016, it concluded that *" the electrode is well-positioned in the middle position and the new pains cannot be driven by peripheral stimulation. He does not think that repositioning is indicated."*

March 10, 2017: Consultation with Doctor R, a neurologist. He proposes a drug trial with Mantadix and Lamictal to relieve the feelings of intense burns and acute pains. Stopping this treatment one month later following an allergic reaction. The pains in the hand are still present and those in the lower back and lower limbs are constantly increasing and without respite.

June 13, 2017: Lumbar bone density test and left hip
Conclusion: *" Bone mineral density is moderately lowered. "*

June 16, 2017: Bone scan.
Conclusion: "*Scintigraphic appearance without arguments for a phase-dependent algodystrophy without elimination of a chronic cold form.*"

Oct 20 and 24, 2017: Consultations with Doctors. R and B, are following a persistent lower limb pain and waking up with pain in the MSD.
Conclusions: "*The situation is still chaotic, no neurological abnormalities; lower extremity pain cannot be related to the electrode or stimulation because they persist even when the device is switched off. Regarding the MSD, a proposal to change pacemaker brand.*"

Oct 30, 2017: Lumbosacral spine scanner.
Conclusions: "*The examination found a L4-L5 disc disease with a protrusive disk overhang a little more marked in the lower part of the left foramen but without the image of disc herniation or disc discord. Degenerative disc disease L5-S1 with a small osteophyte of the lower L5 plateau deforming the lower part of the right foramen.*"

Nov 7, 2017: Consultation at the DAC Poitiers in multidisciplinary with the presence of a neurosurgeon, a pain doctor, a psychologist, and a nurse. The pains are still there ...
Conclusions: "*The problem goes far beyond her right upper limb algodystrophy and is really a patient who has very little non-painful body surface in consultation. It has an overall lowering of the threshold of nociception.*" Support in CAD recommended.

Nov 30, 2017: Consultation with Doctor F, a specialist in pain at the Clinique de la Sauvegarde in Lyon.
Conclusions: "*The examination of the hand is cold, this net change of temperature with respect to the contralateral side. I also note a cutaneous hyperaesthesia not systematized in the painful territory.*" The flexion-extension of the joint is very limited at the level of the fingers. The burns are mostly in the thumb. DN4 positive at the thumb and two feet. Proposed venous blocks.

Dec 7, 2017: Cervical Spine Scanner.
Conclusions: " *Minimal stage desmopathy from C4 to C7. Neurostimulation probe in place.*" In the end, the pain persists, the probe is well-positioned and cannot cause problems in the lower limbs.

2018
Jan 11, 2018: Case change:
The pain was awakened in the MSD and back, Doctor B, proceeded to a change the box. It is now a Boston Spectra rechargeable. This one has clearly lowered the pains, but not of functional return of the hand. Lower limb pain is still present and acute

Jan 23, 2018: EMG of the lower limbs.
Conclusion: RAS

Feb 6, 2018: Consultation with Doctor P, a rheumatologist Lyon Sud Pierre Bénite Hospital
Conclusions: " *The clinical examination of this day found multiple painful points and in particular the 18 points fibromyalgia out of 18. The pains are poorly systematized to correspond to a frank radiculalgie. The bone scintigraphy did not find any notable elements apart from a cold-phase reflex sympathetic appearance of the right hand. I think we can conclude with a table of fibromyalgia complicating the initial algodystrophy.*"

Proposal of spa treatment, balneotherapy, physio, and prosecution care psyche

May 2018: Spa treatment in Lamalou les Bains in rheumatology. Mud baths; poultices; soft gym; jets. No change in pain.

July 24, 2018: Bone scintigraphy

Conclusions: " *MSD stability, discrete hyper fixation of all joints of the left lower limb to the limit of significant.*"

Aug 31, 2018: Consultation with Doctor R who thinks rather of a phenomenon of somatization at the level of the lower limbs and disruption of the central nervous system following my MSD dystrophy.

Sept 05, 2018: Consultation with Doctor JA in internal medicine Lyon Sud which confirms the diagnosis of fibromyalgia with dysregulation of the central nervous system and hypersensitivity with lowering of the nociception threshold.

Sept 2018: Diagnosis left foot dystrophy. Setting up epitomax 50mg at night.

Nov 20, 2018: Diagnosis of cone dystrophy by Doctor G.V. ophthalmologist.

Dec 5, 2018: Kleber Lyon retinal exploration center consultation. Confirmation of the diagnosis of hereditary retinal dystrophy with central retinal involvement.

Since March 2018, I had a venous block on my right hand with tourniquet and injection of xylocaine without any effectiveness.

2019

Jan 22, 2019: Consultation with Professor G at the ophthalmological center of Paris. After examinations, I have no cone dystrophy but Stargardt's disease. He does not understand how this disease could develop so late and especially why my eyesight on the right eye has fallen so quickly (in a few months). Hypotheses: medications taken, venous blocks?

March 28, 2019: Placement of a new electrode placed in T9, T11 for my algodystrophy that migrated from the right arm to the left foot. Hospitalization at the Clinique de la Sauvegarde de Lyon for five days as a complication with leakage of the spinal fluid.

April 23, 2019: Radio control of the laying of the electrode.
Conclusions: "*Stiffness of the cervical spine; Static disturbance with a scoliotic inflexion of the right-convex thoracolumbar spine with rotation of vertebral bodies; L3-L4, L4-L5 and L5-S1 disc disease with posterior disc narrowing and posterior low back lumbar arthrosis.*" There is, therefore, a worsening of the condition of my back since my accident of October 02, 2012.

Nowadays:
The pains this faded at the MSD Grâ that the new neurostimulator. But I still do not find the use of my hand. For the left foot, the sensations of burns, vice, tingling calmed down thanks to the new electrode. However, I still have muscle and joint pain; a feeling of intense tiredness; regular headaches; dizziness; a little restful sleep; difficulties of attention and concentration; visual fatigue... I am always followed by Doctor DS in psychotherapy. I do hypnosis, self-hypnosis, reiki, relaxation, balneotherapy, applications of essential oils, adapted pilates, Qi Gong. But nothing works ...

To note:
Allergies to many molecules. A true intolerance to gluten.

In the family:
Osteoarthritis
Arthritis
Rheumatism
Rhumatismes Psoriatic
Heart problems
Diabetes

Cholesterol
AVC
Colorectal cancer
Glaucoma

Ongoing treatment:
Kardegic 75MG
Doliprane 1g according to the pains
Optimizet continuously
Epitomax 50mg 1 cp evening
Drugs already tested: lyrica,
neurontin, cymbalta, laroxyl, rivotril, mantadix, lamictal, cortisone,
codeine, izalgi, tramadol, lamaline, lidocaine, versatis, deroxat, acupan ...
stop every time because of allergies or major reactions.

Treatments established since Oct 2, 2012

Drugs	Dosage	Start date	End date
Baclofen 4mg	2 cp morning and evening	02.10.12	09.10.12
Tylenol 1g	1 cp 3 times / day	02.10.12	16.10.12
Diclofenac 50 mg	1cp morning and evening	09.10.12	16.10.12
Ibuprofen 400 mg	1 cp 3times / day	19/10/12	12/11/14
Ketoprofen 100 mg	1 cp 3times / day	26.02.12	03/26/13
Lyrica 25mg *	1cp 3times / day	29/11/13	04/01/2015
Lyrica 100mg	1cp in the evening	12/10/13	03/18/14
Lyrica 150mg	1 cp in the evening	04/18/14	01/01/15
Lyrica 200mg	1 cp in the evening	01/01/15	04/01/15
Paxil 20 mg	½ cp at night	05/21/14	01.01.18

Aspirin 75 mg	1 packet in the evening	12/11/14	
Icaz (Isradipine)5mg	1 cp in the evening	12/11/14	01/01/16
Acetaminophen 1g	1cp 3times / day	21/11/14	
Nefopam (Acupan)	On demand	21/11/14	
Amitriptyline 25mg *	5 drops in the evening	23/12/16	04/01/17
Amantadine 100mg *	1 cp morning and noon	03/10/17	04/10/17
Lamictal 100mg *	1 cp morning and evening	03/10/17	04/10/17
Topamax 50mg	1 cp in the evening	01/10/18	03/28/2019

* Discontinuation of these drugs due to drug intolerance.

For eyes

Indobiotic UD and Sterdex in both eyes for eight days from March 27, 2017 to April 04, 2017. Thealose and Naabak two times a day from April 05, 2017 to September 2018.

Infiltration performed on Oct 5, 2013

Infiltration under ultrasound with pre anesthesia xylocaine half-bulb diprostène in trapezo metacarpal and right half- bulb diprostène entitled sesamoid.

Venous block 2018

Realization of six venous blocks IV right-hand xylocaine 1% 15 ml under tourniquet inflated to 200 mm/Hg on the following dates:
03/20/18, 04/24/18, 06/01/18, 09/07/18, 08/20/18, 09/24/18.

Reaction to each block with sensations of nausea, head-turning, feeling of coming out of general anesthesia, lips sleeping for about 24-hours.

LIVING WITH COMPLEX REGIONAL PAIN SYNDROME (CRPS):

MY THIRTY-FOUR YEARS OF NERVE BLOCKS, PAIN MEDICATIONS, AND SURGERIES

By: Eric M. Phillips

My complex regional pain syndrome (CRPS) formerly called reflex sympathetic dystrophy (RSD) story started on December 7, 1985, after a car accident. I was 20-years old then. I was two months shy of my 21st birthday. It was a Friday night, and a classmate from high school had stopped by my parent's house. It was around 10:00 pm when my friend showed up. He asked me if I wanted to go hang out with him and his girlfriend. Since I was young and had nothing to do on a Friday night, I decided to go for a ride. Little did I know that taking that ride would change my life forever.

I remember that night like it was yesterday. It was a cold December night; we had a little dusting of snow on the ground enough to make the car slide a little while driving. We had about a 30-minute drive from my parent's house to my friends' girlfriend's house. We were not too far from our destination, when all of a sudden, I noticed that the driver started to speed up. He was doing about 55-mph in a 25-mph zone. Before I knew what was going on the car went off the road, and we hit a rock monument on my side of the car. Before the impact, I braced myself. I pushed my left foot into the floorboard. At impact, I felt an electrical jolt travel up my left leg, and I heard and felt a pop in my lower back. I also hit my shoulder on the dashboard and hit my head on the windshield. I was knocked out for a minute from hitting my head on the windshield. When I came too, I noticed the driver was knocked out, big time! He had hit his head on the steering wheel. There was blood everywhere.

When the EMT's showed up at the scene, I remember trying to get out of the car. I was unable to do that since the passenger side door was crushed in. So, the EMT had to pull me out of the car over the driver who was still knocked out. The EMT placed me in the back seat of the car. The impact of the crash was so bad that it threw my glasses into the back seat. I was lucky to find them.

While the EMT was placing me on a stretcher, he asked me if I was in any pain. At that time, I only had a little pain. He said to me "wait until you wake up in the morning you will feel the pain." Boy! He was he right! I was in so much pain. Little did I know that the pain in my foot and leg was CRPS.

While I was in the ER I was asked by the nurse if I knew how many drinks my friend had that night? She informed me that he was over the legal drinking limit. I know my friend was a heavy drinker at times. The only thing I knew was what he told me. He said he had a lot of drinks at lunchtime and after work. He was the type that could drink a lot and still function in life. When he arrived at my parent's house, he seemed fine. I guess that the amount of alcohol that was still in his system made him pass out while he was driving. The irony is that I did not have any drinks that night. Maybe if I did my body would have been more relaxed and maybe I would have not been as hurt as I was. My friend only got some stitches in his head. I got a lifetime worth of pain.

My Diagnosis

After I was released from the emergency room, I went home to sleep it off. I remember waking up in so much pain. I had to wait to see my Orthopedic doctor on Monday morning. The only thing this doctor did for me was to refer me to physical therapy and told me to see him in three weeks. This treatment went on for about six months. As, time went on, my pain got worse.

After six months of not receiving any help from this Orthopedic doctor. I went to seek answers from other doctors, such as other Orthopedic doctors, and Neurologist. I must have seen over 20-30 doctors over a two-and-a-half-year span. No one could give me an answer to my pain problem. I remember some doctors telling me the pain was all in my head. I am sure many CRPS patients have heard the same line from a few doctors.

In the late spring/early summer of 1987, I went to see a Vascular doctor at the Mass General Hospital (MGH). Doctor D.B., performed a few vascular tests on my left foot and leg. He came to the conclusion that I might have RSD (back, then they called it RSD, not CRPS) He then recommended that I make an appointment to see a pain specialist, Doctor D.C. also from the MGH pain clinic to see if I was suffering from RSD. I went to see Doctor D.C. for my first, nerve block to help confirm the diagnosis of RSD. The results of the nerve block did confirm I had RSD-CRPS. Thank you, Doctor D.C. and Doctor D.B.! I was finally diagnosed with CRPS. I finally got a name to what was causing my pain. I remember talking with my parents, we all said RSD? What the hell is that? Well, we got a crash course on what RSD-CRPS was. I was finally on the right path to learning what RSD-CRPS was and what life had in store for me....

After being diagnosed by Doctor D.C., he requested that I obtain all my medical records from the Orthopedic doctor that I first saw after my accident. After receiving my medical records from the doctor, my parents and I started to read the records. It came to our surprise that this doctor wrote in his last note before he released me from his care that I had a mild case of RSD. Wow! We were all shocked that he never said anything to me.

What gets me upset is he never informed me of my diagnosis. I wish he would have said to me "hey Eric, I think you have this condition called RSD, but I do not know a lot about it." He could have said "Eric, I can either refer you to someone who treats the condition, or you can pursue another doctor who can help you." That never happened! It would have been nice to have known what I had and maybe get some early treatment and try to put this into remission.

After my diagnosis, I started to do research on RSD/CRPS to help educate myself. I spent countless hours in the medical library in my local area to find medical articles on RSD. Over time, I amassed hundreds of medical articles on this awful condition. I also started to search for others who suffered from CRPS. I remember finding a young woman near my age who lived in the same city that I did. After meeting and talking with her, I found out that we saw the same doctor. She like me had CRPS in her left leg. She was also misdiagnosed by the same doctor. She also went searching for years for a proper diagnosis too. In addition, she found in her medical records that the doctor noted she had a mild case of RSD, but he never informed her. Nice doctor! It's sad that he knew the diagnosis and never said anything to either of us.

Treatment and Surgeries

The road to dealing with CRPS leads you to many forms of treatments and surgeries (in some cases). In my case, I started to develop a deformity in my left foot, ankle, and toes. This deformity baffled many doctors during my quest to get a proper diagnosis. I remember one Neurologist telling me that I had dystonia and not RSD. Little did this doctor know that some cases of RSD-CRPS can develop a dystonic posture or deformity. This issue was my case. I guess that I am lucky to have a deformity (in some ways). It was a visual thing that someone could look at it and say that must be painful. Most CRPS patients do not develop any type of deformity, which should not discount their pain.

In the beginning, after my diagnosis, I had many sympathetic nerve blocks, bier blocks (which are one of the most painful types of block anyone could ever go through). You count every millisecond; it is unbearable pain. I did two of these to prove a point that they don't work. I must have been crazy at that time, Lol!

Going into my third year of suffering from CRPS, the deformity in my left foot was getting worse. It got so bad that the joints in my great toe (big toe) froze. On, December 14, 1988, I had my first surgery. I had a fusion of the left great toe. This surgery was done at the MGH by my Orthopedic, Doctor J.J... Two months, after the surgery my CRPS started to spread up my left leg above my knee. The pain got so bad I was no longer able to put pressure or weight on my left leg (I lost the use of my leg). So, for the next 20 plus years, I went around on crutches and used a wheelchair for long-distance.

Since then, after my first foot surgery, I went for more nerve blocks to help control the pain. These nerve blocks did not help too much, until I met Doctor Hooshang Hooshmand of Vero Beach, Florida. His blocks gave me the best relief. Read more about Doctor Hooshmand further on in this story.

Over the past thirty-four years of dealing with CRPS, I have had hundreds of epidural nerve blocks, trigger point injections, SI joint injections and so on... Sometimes, I had some relief from the blocks and sometimes not. Most patients have been through the same thing over time. It's a part of dealing with this disease and dealing with doctors who don't understand the disease or know how to treat it. Sometimes, these treatments work, and there are times when nothing helps with the pain.

The other part of my injury from the car accident was my back. I herniated a few discs at the L-5/S-1 level of my lower spine. It took me three years after my accident to find a doctor who knew about back issues and CRPS. I was fortunate to meet an Orthopedic spine specialist Doctor P.B. from the Dartmouth Hitchcock Medical Center in Lebanon NH.

I found Doctor P.B. through an article he wrote on RSD associated with low lumbar disc herniation. He performed two back surgeries on me. On, July 10, 1991, I had my first of three back surgeries. The first back surgery helped my back for a short time.

I had my second back surgery on October 27, 2004, which was the same day the Boston Red Sox won their first World Series in 86-years. I will never forget that day! Once again, this second back surgery did not help for too long either.

Now jumping to October 23rd and 24th, 2017, I had my third and final back surgery done by Doctor P.G. from Boston. This time, I had to have spinal fusion surgery at the L-4, L-5, S-1 levels. This surgery was brutal. They cut me in my abdomen, and my lower back to install the cages, rods, and screws that are now a part of my spine.

This surgery helped with some of my back pain, but it has left me with some other issues, including SI joint pain. After having this type of surgery, I said to myself, no more back surgery for this kid!

To understand how CRPS can change a person's life, one must see the physical changes that my foot and leg went through over 23-years. These pictures below show the stages of how my foot and leg changed over the years. These pictures will show you the deformities which affected my toes, ankle, the skin changes that took place over the years, and the infections I had in my foot and toes for over a year and a half.

My Amputation

The most difficult surgery that I went through in my life was on August 25th and 27th 2008. I had to have a two-stage amputation. I had to have this surgery because I battled with infections in my left foot and leg for over a year and a half. The infections first started on February 14, 2007(Happy Valentine's Day!). I was admitted to the hospital monthly to a month and a half to help fight these infections with I.V. Antibiotics which did not do too much for the infections and made me feel like crap. In June of 2008, I was in the hospital again for a week to treat the infections. After being in the hospital for a week, my doctors came into my hospital room to discuss with me that the Antibiotics were not working to help control the infections. They discussed with me my options of what to do next. They said I could return monthly for the next five to six months and do more I.V. Antibiotic treatment until the infection kills you or we can do an amputation. Boy, that was a big-time wake-up call to hear the word's AMPUTATION! Wow! I said to my primary care physician (Doctor P.G. from the MGH) I have to think about that for a minute. He recommended that I should speak with a vascular surgeon from MGH who does amputations.

I told Doctor P.G., that I would agree to speak with this surgeon Doctor M.C., also from the MGH in Boston. He was such a great guy and a great surgeon.

He spent over an hour with me going over my options and discussing the pros and cons of doing this procedure. I had many questions for him regarding my CRPS. I asked the typical questions like do you know what CRPS is? How many patients have you seen with the disease? Have you performed an amputation on CRPS patients before and what were the results? Well, he was honest with me and told me he knew about CRPS, but he never did an amputation on a patient with CRPS. I told him my hopes and fears of doing this surgery. He was open to learning more about CRPS and amputations. This impressed me to know he was willing to learning more about what I was dealing with.

After meeting with Doctor M.C., and going home, I took the month to beat myself up (mentally) with deciding to do the surgery to amputate my left leg above the knee. I spoke with all my family, friends, and other relatives about what I was planning on having done. I also spoke with a wonderful Psychologist Doctor B (as I call her). She helped me so much in dealing with the fact of having an amputation. She put it in the best perspective to me. She had asked me if my foot and leg were my friend or enemy in this time of my life? My answer to her was that it was my enemy; after that conversation, I made my decision to do the surgery. Thank you, Doctor B!

One week, before my surgery, I met with Doctor M.C., to discuss what we were going to do for the surgery. At, this point and time the infections were at their worst. I was only sleeping between one to two hours a night due to the pain of the CRPS and the infections. Once, Doctor M.C., saw how bad the infections got, he said that he had to rethink what route he was going to take for my surgery. He said since the infections got worse, he had to do a two-stage amputation. As he explained to me that on the first day, he would amputate my foot at the ankle to let the rest of the infection drain out of my leg for a day. He then asked me if I wanted to stay awake for this first surgery which would be a guillotine cut of the foot at the ankle. He said it would only take 10 minutes for the procedure. I asked him if he was smoking crack in his pipe? Lol! I told him a big NO! I wanted to be knocked the hell out for the surgery. Well, I must say that the first part of my amputation surgery went well. To be honest, I felt great not having that infected and painful (for over 20 plus years) foot on my body anymore. I was like a different person laughing and telling jokes to the nurses and doctors. So, on the third day of being in the hospital, I had the second stage of the amputation done. The surgery went well, but I felt more pain then I had after the first surgery. I knew that it was not going to be an easy ride without having some type of pain.

I was in the hospital for six days. I remember the first time I tried to get out of bed without having my leg. It felt strange, but I was used to not using my left leg to walk for the past 20 plus years, so it was no big deal getting used to being an amputee. I was released from the hospital and went home to finally get some well-deserved rest. As one knows, no one sleeps while they are in the hospital. This fact is because the nurses need to check your blood pressure, draw blood or give you meds rather than let you sleep between the hours of 1 A.M. and 6 A.M. I was also looking forward to getting some good home-cooked food from my mom. You know how hospital food can be.

Well, my first night home sleeping in my bed did not go as well as I planned. The moment I got into my bed, I started to get really bad muscle spasms in my stump (which was nicknamed Stumpy by my dear friend Tracey P.).

These spasms lasted six to seven hours. I could not move an inch in my bed without having severe pain in my stump from the spasms. I called my surgeon's office and I spoke with a doctor who was covering for him over the weekend. I told him what was going on and asked him to phone in a prescription for a muscle relaxant. He said that I have to drive back the hospital in Boston to be checked out. I said to him are you crazy. I knew what is going on, and I needed something for the spasms. So, I hung up the phone since I was not getting anywhere with this idiot doctor. I asked my mom to call 911 to take me to the local ER. They came right away and took me to the local hospital. After being there for 6-hours, they sent me home with a prescription for a muscle relaxant. It did help with the spasms briefly, so I was able to get some sleep.

The next night, the same thing happened to me again. The spasms started back up again. After a few hours of dealing with this again, I asked my wonderful mother to call 911 again to take me back to the MGH in Boston again to see my surgeon to learn what was going on with all these spasms. Well, the reason for all these spasms was due to another infection that I developed above my incision. After finding this out, I was back on I.V. Antibiotics for another six days. Thank God that the Antibiotics helped with the infection this time. It was well worth staying in the hospital again for another six days.

Finally, I was home and resting in my bed again. Then the fun started with adjusting to my new life of being an amputee with CRPS. For weeks my days were filled with visiting nurses coming in to change the dressings on my stump (stumpy) and checking for any new infections. Thank God I never had another bad infection again. Knock on wood! After a few weeks of being home, I started in-home physical therapy (PT). It was fun learning new ways to do things as an amputee. I was ahead of the game because I lived the past 20 plus years of not using my left leg due to the pain, so I was used to using crutches and a wheelchair.

After about a month of in-home PT I started out-patient PT at a local place not too far from my home. This is where I started to build up my strength again to get ready to be fitted for my first prosthetic. In, October of 2008 I started the process of being fitted for my first prosthetic socket and microprocessor knee (C-Leg) I gave my new leg a nickname. I call him Lefty. I did not realize how much work goes into making a prosthetic socket. You have to go through a casting process to have a mold of your stump so they can start creating your socket. It is a very amazing process to witness. I was very fortunate to be referred to Nextstep Bionics and Prosthetics in Warwick, RI (I won't name names; you know who you are Lol!). All of the great people at Nextstep have given me my life back with my new leg.

On November 12, 2008, I took my first steps walking after 20-plus years of only walking on one leg. It was a scary feeling taking my first steps on my new prosthetic leg. I felt like Forest Gump! Run Forest Run! I had no clue what I was doing, but I did it. I think it was my Dad watching over me that day.

I just wish he was there to see me walking in person. I remember the look on my mom's face when she saw me take my first steps. It was the best thing to see! I saw how happy she was. It made me feel great to see her so happy.

Most people do not know that being an amputee, we are constantly going through changes with the anatomy of our stumps. I was told in the first year of being an amputee that I may go through at least three to six different sockets. Well, I was lucky I only went through three sockets in my first year. In total, I have had nine sockets and four knees. I received my fourth new knee (a C-Leg 4) on May 28, 2019. As I tell people it's not easy being an amputee. It can be very painful at times and it can be very challenging and frustrating at times too. It's a lot of work walking on a prosthetic leg for many people, including myself.

The fun part of having my sockets made is that they can take any T-shirt with a design on it and laminate it to the socket. It's a cool process to watch. I have had many cool designs on my sockets over the years. Most people who know me, know that I am a big Todd Rundgren Fan. He is my favorite music artist. I have been following his music since my older brother Michael turned me on to Todd's music in the 1970s. I have had many of Todd's concert T-shirt images on my sockets over the years. Todd has been so kind as to autograph a few of my sockets when I have met him at his concerts.

Well, I must tell you that having CRPS and being an amputee can be very difficult to deal with at times. As I tell patients who have called or emailed me; that they are thinking about having their arm or leg amputated. I tell them that it is a long hard process to think about and a difficult decision to make.

First off, there are many factors that you have to take into consideration before you get to the point of amputation. You must exhaust all your options (other treatments) before doing an amputation. Typically having an amputation will not cure your CRPS. Sometimes, it can cause more pain and spread of the disease.

Sometimes, people think that if you cut the affected CRPS limb off you are going to be pain-free. This is not the case for most people who go through this procedure. There is an article written by a group of doctors from the Netherlands who have reported that only 1% of the CRPS population can wear a prosthetic limb after amputation. I am glad that I am a part of the 1% of a group that can wear it.

In my case, I had an above-knee amputation (way above, my left knee). I had a long discussion with my surgeon Doctor M.C. about how far above the knee we were going to amputate? I was grateful that Doctor M.C. trusted me in my decision of where we should amputate. I went a few inches above the line of discoloration from the CRPS, which was past my mid-thigh. I have been told by my doctors and prosthetist that I made the right decision on the level that I had chosen.

The most difficult part of dealing with being an amputee is having phantom limb pain (PLP). Boy, I found out the hard way. To be honest PLP is more painful than CRPS pain. I have had to deal with PLP since my surgery, and I still have it after 11-years. The pain that I feel when the phantom pain hits is a feeling of being repeatedly stabbed in my stump. It's a painful feeling that I would not wish on anyone. People say to me that your leg is gone, how come you still have a feeling that your foot and leg are still there? When they do an amputation, they don't remove the nerves that were connected from your foot, ankle, and leg to your brain. They don't remove the nerves (it's not like a wiring harness in a car that you can remove. Lol!). The nerves that were connected to my foot and leg are still in my residual limb (my stump). These nerves are still connected to my brain, which is the reason why I can still feel my old limb. To this day I can still feel the screw that was in my great toe and I still feel the infections that I had on my foot and toes. This is a very strange feeling, to say the least!

There are many nights when the phantom pain comes and it can stay with me for days. The longest that I went without sleep due to the PLP was 38-

hours. I can always tell when the "Phantom" (as I call him) is coming to visit me. The change of weather can cause the "Phantom" to rear its ugly head at times.

My honest recommendation to any CRPS patient who is thinking about having an amputation is to think long and hard about doing it. As in my case, I had no choice about doing this surgery.

The infections that were caused by my CRPS were affecting my health and my life. My decision came down to life or limb, so I picked life over my limb.

There has only been one time in the past 11-years that I said, I regretted having the amputation. It was on my first night home after being released from the hospital. This was when I had the brutal spasms in my stump for over six to seven hours. Since that night, I have not regretted my decision at all. Once, we got everything under control, I started looking forward to walking again and starting my life over.

If you are at that point in your life and at the stage of having CRPS that you have to amputate, please take the time to talk with your doctors, family, friends, and a good Psychologist before you make that final decision. Also, do some soul searching too. It's a big procedure to go through and a long road ahead of you living as an amputee atop of living with CRPS. Please talk with someone who has been through this surgery. It will help you in many ways.

I was lucky to speak with someone with CRPS that went through having an amputation of their left leg. This person helped me in so many ways. Thank you, Lou M., for being such a great friend and for being there for me during my surgery.

Medications

Medications are a big part of dealing with CRPS. There are so many types of medications out there to help you deal with the pain of CRPS. In my case, some medications do not agree with me. On November 17, 1997, I was having a procedure done on my leg so I could be cast for a new brace for my left leg, to help with the deformity that I had developed due to the CRPS. I was at Doctor Hooshmand's office having a nerve block done to help with the pain of getting cast for the brace. I was on three different medications at that time I was on Klonopin, Baclofen, and Buprenex (Buprenorphine). Unfortunately, this event was the day that I had an allergic reaction to these medications.

One thing I do remember on that day was being in the procedure room and I was getting hot and tired. I was fortunate that my friend Debra was in the room with me, while I was having my leg cast for the new brace. She noticed that I was turning blue and I had stopped breathing. It was the worst thing you could fear. I had gone into respiratory failure.

I had no clue what was going on at that time. Debra was able to get Doctor Hooshmand and others into the room to help me. They called 911 to get me to the local hospital.

From what I was told, they had to jump-start my heart, and they rushed me to the emergency room. I remember waking up from one of the best sleeps that I have ever had in my life. The only thing that I can remember is that it was dark and peaceful. I did not see any bright lights or angels. I do not remember knowing what was going on or where I was. When I was looking around the room to see where I was, I then saw Doctor Hooshmand standing on the left-hand side of me. Once I saw him, I knew that I was safe.

During the event of having respiratory failure I had aspirated, and I developed Aspiration Pneumonia. Great another thing to add to my list of problems that day. After coming through all the day's events, I was admitted to the hospital for a week. We do not know which of the three medications may have caused the allergic reaction which caused the respiratory failure.

To this day, I no longer take any of these medications. I would rather be safe than sorry. I would never want to go through that ordeal again in my life.

On that note. I am left with taking very few medications. The few medications that I can tolerate are Ultracet and Dilaudid for pain and anti-inflammatories such as Mobic, and Diclofenac. I am very lucky to have such a high pain threshold. Oh, lucky me!

Once, again from the bottom of my heart, I am very grateful to everyone who helped save my life that day. I am one very lucky guy!

Starting an RSD-CRPS Support Group

Over time, I started to meet many others who also suffer from CRPS. In the early 1990s, I started a local RSD support group with a few other patients that I met after my diagnosis.

As support groups go, people come and go. I was the only one running the group after some time. I would hold meetings at a local hospital in my area. Over time, the group got bigger, and we started to get patients to come to our meeting from out of state. I would get doctors, physical therapist, and lawyers to speak to the group. These lectures were helpful to many patients, including me. To know that you are not alone dealing with such a painful disease was the best medicine for me. Running the group or just talking with another patient on the phone has helped me cope with my pain and to know that each one of us is just another piece to the puzzle we call CRPS.

Through running the group, I have been fortunate to meet so many wonderful and brave people. Some of these amazing people have become close and lifetime friends of mine.

Even, though I no longer run the local support group I have kept in touch with many of the people that I met through the support group.

After the local support group meetings ended, I started a website www.rsdinfo.com to help educate others suffering from CRPS. From my website, I have received tens of thousands of e-mails from patients from around the world.

Instead of meeting at a local place to talk about CRPS, I now do it through e-mail or by phone. I enjoy talking to patients, and I love trying to help them someway either by giving them a referral to a doctor, lawyer, therapist in their local area or just to be the one to tell them that they are not alone. It helps me to help others.

Doctor Hooshang Hooshmand

In 1993, I was so very fortunate to meet the late Doctor Hooshang Hooshmand (or as I call him Doctor Hoosh). I met him through the textbook he wrote about RSD. It was the most interesting and helpful book I have ever read on the topic of RSD-CRPS. After reading the first few pages of his book, I picked up the phone and called his office. He was so kind as to take my call. He spent over an hour on the phone with me. I was so impressed he took the time to speak with me. After talking with him and reading his book, it seemed we shared the same philosophy regarding RSD-CRPS.

He was the first doctor that I had ever talked with who shared the same views I had on treating this disease. After our first phone conversation, I invited Doctor Hooshmand to speak to our local RSD-CRPS support group.

He was so gracious to accept my invitation. He took the time out of his busy schedule to fly to Massachusetts and give a lecture to our support group. He was a great speaker, and he took the time to explain things to the patients.

He also took time after his lecture to personally speak with every patient in the room. There are a few things that I remember about that day. During Doctor Hooshmand's lecture, he said two things that have stuck with me over the years.

First, he told the group that "the people who know the most about CRPS are not the doctors, it is the patients who have the most knowledge about the condition because they are the ones who live with the pain every day." The other thing he said was, "do you know what the difference is between God and a doctor? He said that God does not think he is a doctor, but most doctors think they are Gods." These two statements are so true.

I was so impressed he said these things to our group. I finally met a doctor who got it! He was someone who knew about this disease and knew how to treat it. He also treated his CRPS patients with the utmost respect.

Over the time of knowing Doctor Hooshmand, he had come to speak to our support group often. In 1995, Doctor Hooshmand asked me to work with him to construct a large-scale RSD-CRPS conference for both patients and physicians. This conference format was one of the first of its kind. We had both patients and physicians attending the conference at the same venue. The conference was such a success, we decided to do two more conferences with the same format for patients and physicians in 1997 and 2000.

After our first conference together, Doctor Hooshmand asked me to help him write some medical articles that were published in medical journals. I agreed to help and work with him. I also developed a website www.rsdrx.com for Doctor Hooshmand to help educate both CRPS patients and the medical community. This work was one of the best things to happen in my life besides getting married last year (2018) to my beautiful and loving wife Mercedes.

Working on dozens of RSD-CRPS articles with Doctor Hooshmand has helped me gain so much knowledge about this disease. Doctor Hooshmand is a great teacher and mentor. More than being a great mentor, he became a great friend to me. I am so blessed and grateful that I had the honor to meet and work with one of the greatest Neurologist that has ever treated RSD-CRPS.

As, I say to all my friends, family, and other CRPS patients that I am the luckiest guy in the world to do what I have done in my lifetime, to work with such a great man who has helped so many people worldwide.

Besides working with Doctor Hooshmand, I also received treatment from him. He treated my CRPS and lower back issues up until his retirement. His nerve blocks worked the best for me. His treatments helped me manage my pain which, gave me a better quality of life.

Once again, I am most grateful to the late Doctor Hooshmand for treating my pain and helping other patients for over 40-years. What impressed me most about Doctor Hooshmand was his compassion and tireless efforts to help his patients who were suffering from the chronic pain of RSD. In my opinion, he was the Archangel of RSD for helping so many patients. He always tried to provide his patients with a better quality of life. He was truly an amazing man, physician, mentor, and best friend.

Conclusion: Living life with CRPS

Living the past 34-years with a chronic pain condition we call CRPS has not been an easy journey for me. CRPS is a complex disease that can change a person's life in minutes, may it be from an injury or surgery.

From the moment that I was in my accident, it placed me on a different path in life. I had no idea which direction this path was taking me on. I am so glad my life took this path, it has helped me cope and learn about CRPS, and it also put me on a path to help others with CRPS.

From the time of my accident to the time of my diagnosis I had never heard of reflex sympathetic dystrophy (RSD) which is the former name of CRPS (I still like to call it RSD). Once I was diagnosed and had a name to my problem as I called it, I felt a sense of relief that I knew I was not crazy and the pain that I felt in my left foot and leg was real and it was not in my head as some doctors in the past had mentioned to me.

My path of CRPS has shown me that I was never alone. First off, I am very fortunate to have the best support system from my mother, Janet and my late father Lenny, my two older brothers, Michael and Keith, and their families, all my relatives, and my best friends in the world Mike I. and Jimmy H. Without all their support, I would not be the person that I am today. Over the past six years, I have been truly blessed to have met the love of my life, my wife Mercedes. Mercedes and her three children and her grandson have been so supportive of me, through all the ups and downs that I have been through in my life.

Many patients ask me how do I cope with living with this pain? I tell them what has gotten me through the past 34-years of living with CRPS. The first thing that helps me cope with dealing with CRPS and being an amputee is the support that I receive from my wonderful family and friends. The other things that help me cope with the pain are listening to my favorite music artist Todd Rundgren (my bio-feedback) and having humor in my life. I tell other patients that I always try to find some humor in dealing with my pain. I feel if I don't laugh, I will cry.

All patients must have some type of support system in place. It does not matter if their support comes from their immediate family or close friends. This type of support is a key component to help patients deal with such a complex and painful disease such as CRPS.

If a patient lacks family or friends to receive support from, there are other alternatives that they can look into. Today, patients can find many online

CRPS support groups they can join on many social media networks. These groups can be helpful to patients who do not have family or friends to give them support.

CRPS is a disease that affects so many people worldwide. It changes a person's life, physically, mentally, socially and financially. It can ruin a person's life.

The sad thing about the car accident that I was in, is that the so-called friend of mine that I was driving with thought the car accident was a joke. It was no joke! Since that accident, I have lived the past 34-years in chronic pain from developing CRPS, dealing with my back issues, and all the surgeries that I had to endure over the years. Over the past 34-years, I have yet to hear from this so-called friend. He has never called to reach out to me to see how I am doing. I guess he has to live with himself for the rest of his life for what happened to me? I have moved on with my life and I am grateful that I was not killed in the accident.

My path of living with CRPS has made me grow as a man. CRPS has taught me to learn about my condition, help educate myself, and to help others who are dealing with the same disabling painful condition.

I have been fortunate for the path that CRPS has taken me on. It has given me the opportunity to meet so many wonderful people with CRPS, meet Doctor Hooshmand and work with him on many important CRPS projects that I hope has helped many patients over the years.

RSD AND ME
By: Anita Boyer

My life dramatically changed after a sprain/strain injury to my right shoulder on April 17, 1998. In preparation of a move from one office location to another, I picked up a "banker's" box of Pendaflex files, which I thought my 5′ 3″, 110-pound body was strong enough to lift. In hindsight, I should have left that up to the various male supervisors standing in the office with me. After picking up the box, I realized immediately that it was much heavier than I thought and while my hands were still in the right-side holes of the box, the box fell to the ground. My left hand instinctively came out of the box, but I heard a pop in the right shoulder. Because I worked for the mayor's office in my city, you don't leave unless you are literally dying, and it was approximately eleven in the morning. My direct supervisor was in attendance at the time and instructed me to visit a nearby hospital at the end of the day, which was about six that evening, where I was diagnosed with a sprain/strain of the acromioclavicular joint.

I was a single mother of three children, ages ranging from ten to fifteen years old, and was a recent host family for exchange students from other countries (Germany, Norway, and Spain). In July 1998, I had planned a vacation for me and my children to visit three of the exchange students with their families in Germany and Spain. However, in June, my shoulder was rearing the ugliness of a future diagnosis of Reflex Sympathetic Dystrophy (RSD). The pain was getting worse, and my arm was swollen and turning black and blue down to my fingertips. I visited my PCP the end of June, 1998, and he referred me to an orthopedic surgeon who ordered an MRI and told me that he didn't know what was going on, but he didn't like it and that I should cancel my vacation that was to start the very next week. Of course, I told him that I had non-refundable tickets for me and my three children; and that there was no way, after all the planning, I could cancel. He then put my arm in a shoulder binder, which is a sling combined with a band that completely entraps the arm next to the body, so it is of no use.

My job entailed meetings with various Daimler-Chrysler, Jeep, city officials, and railroad companies in our attempt to KEEP JEEP in Toledo, Ohio. As such, a groundbreaking ceremony was originally scheduled during my time in Europe on vacation. Luckily, they changed the groundbreaking to accommodate my vacation schedule until I returned back to work. Although in the end, I still missed it because after arriving home. I went to my local grocery store to resupply my now empty refrigerator only to suffer from a horrific muscle spasm when grabbing a head of lettuce. The next morning it was still so bad that I had to visit the ER and was given Vicodin and Flexeril. Amazingly, I called a colleague and he picked me up and drove me to work that same day. I was apparently high as a kite because my boss stated I could "fly home." I remember sitting at the computer with my five-year-old daughter after taking one of the Vicodin pills. The next thing I remember, I woke up in the ICU of a hospital. Now I'm in the hospital and missing the groundbreaking they rescheduled just for me, I wasn't happy at all about that. It was during this stay that I suffered a small stroke and received my first stellate ganglion block which was used both as a treatment modality and diagnostic as well. However, it wasn't successful as I didn't feel any different before or after the procedure. I also started physical therapy to gain strength back in my right leg (the right arm was already weakened before the stroke).

The year continued to spiral downwards and after seeking help from my PCP once again. This time, he referred me to a chiropractor who started "adjustments" after an X-ray and diagnosis of "lordosis" of the neck. I reluctantly continued for six weeks until I could no longer endure the pain, I felt which only worsened after each visit. The doctor also admitted that I was not doing better and felt that I needed to go in a different direction. This is when I was referred to a neurosurgeon (it's now August of 1998) who ordered a myelogram and I had to deal with a spinal headache and subsequent blood patch to fix this new problem. She also ordered physical therapy (PT) which eventually was canceled by the therapist because I went downhill... fast! He couldn't even touch me anymore without me screaming in pain. The neurosurgeon originally felt it might be thoracic outlet syndrome (TOS) but came to realize more likely it was RSD and referred me to a physiatrist in December of 1998. After being fitted with my shoulder harness, because he claimed I was predestined for RSD due to being loosely jointed, and of course more PT, he made a call that changed my life. He called me in January 1999, to inform me that I had appointments on February 5, 1999 at Cleveland Clinic with several doctors.

The day arrived for my one-day physician-binge, including doctors from pain management (Doctor S.H.), neurology, psychiatry, and physical therapy. I was told that I was a great candidate for their pain program. To this day, I still believe that it was more of a brainwashing program than anything else. I received a call from my physiatrist who told me that I was indeed "enrolled" as an in-patient of the Cleveland Clinic pain management program at the Walker Building. I was so excited initially thinking I would be finally getting the help I needed to get rid of this awful pain. I secured a room at a local hotel the night before. I had successfully kicked my smoking habit six months prior, but was once again a smoker when I checked out. There was so much noise outside my door (next to the elevators on my floor) all night long that I couldn't sleep, and found my way down to the lobby and a vending machine filled with cigarettes, so I bought a pack (back then it was $4 a pack). By the time I arrived at CCF, I had a full-blown migraine due to lack of sleep and smoking.

Upon arriving, the nurses took all my medications...Poof! Gone! I had to fill out a questionnaire rating and describing my pain only to be told that I could NOT mention the "P" word – PAIN -- while in this program. That didn't make a lot of sense to me since that is exactly why I was there in the first place. I couldn't say I felt "pain", but rather I felt "irritated", or "angry", or "sad", etc…you get my drift.   But what I did feel was just that…UNRELENTING PAIN! This was going to be an all-day affair and I met a lot of people with various diagnoses…from scleroderma to PTSD, and everything in between. No one else was there with RSD unfortunately for me. The nurse ushered me into a conference room where I was immediately uneasy because the conference table was surrounded by a medical staff of some sort, but I didn't as of yet recognize everyone. I was introduced to therapists—both occupational and physical—a psychiatrist, nurses, and a biofeedback specialist, as I recall. Fluorescent lights, a phone on the table ringing constantly, and my migraine were not a great combination at all. The psychiatrist (I learned to despise and referred to as "Doctor God") introduced himself and asked who diagnosed me with migraines. I answered, "my neurologist" dumbfounded as could be, to which he replied, "you don't have migraines." Boom! Just like that, I was undiagnosed by a doctor who didn't know me from Adam! What an egocentric narcissist, I thought! And in time, I discovered I wasn't wrong.

I had to describe my history of employment from the time I was sixteen to the present. In my case, I worked undercover for the Vice Squad in my city for a spell. The details I can't discuss, but believe me, I was very glad when it was over. But for some reason, "Doctor God" thought I MUST be lying. Why in the world would I? I had no reason to lie! I was here for what I thought was the reduction of pain in my right arm! It was during this interrogation that I had reached a pivotal part of my migraine and his denial of same – I began vomiting. Suddenly "Doctor God" is asking someone to shut off the lights and remove the incessantly-ringing phone from the room. NOW he believes me, I thought! I had to puke in front of him before he did though.

During this first week, I would arrive at 8:00 a.m. for breakfast with the others in the program, followed by check-in with the nurses for our daily questionnaire, physical therapy, occupational therapy and ending with group therapy. On Fridays, family members were required to attend because they wanted to see if any of us had been "enabled" by other family members. I told them before I even started the program that I didn't have anyone who would drive almost three hours each way to sit in a group therapy session and discuss any problems. I offered two family members who agreed to speak by phone to medical personnel to answer any questions they may have, and they allowed this. I had a hard time with the "enabling" accusation as my situation was a mom to three under-age children. Did they seriously think THEY could be enabling ME? HA! What a joke. By the end of the first week, I left. I certainly didn't need their judging on top of my loss of self-worth as a mom because of this disease. My departure was the direct result of the weird dichotomy of treatment – one side of the hall was treating the pain of the disease and the other side of the hall did everything they could to deny any "feeling" of the "P" word altogether.

The final straw to me leaving so fast was because I had been scheduled for another stellate ganglion block (SGB) with Doctor S.H... Doctor S.H., was one of the premiere RSD physicians in the world who traveled constantly to speak about the diagnosis and treatment of RSD. I am eternally grateful for meeting him when I did, and as a worker's compensation case, was instrumental in receiving my awards. At my first visit, he took extra time and fit me into the schedule to receive an SGB which was the first successful block I had received. As previously stated, the first SGB I had, didn't seem to work. He not only proved I had RSD, but had successfully (or thought magically) made my pain non-existent after the SGB. His explanation for that was that the doctors here didn't block in the right spot to afford the same response. I remember exactly how it felt – it was like my cold arm had switched from the right to the left arms instantly. I had temperature gauges on both thumbs so he could see that it worked as well. I discovered for a successful diagnosis and block, the temperature difference between the affected and non-affected extremity must be three degrees Celsius. I also discovered that I initially had a diagnosis of possible conversion disorder versus RSD, which was now undeniably proven to be RSD.

After the initial SGB wore off, I was instructed to make another appointment for a subsequent SGB from Doctor S.H. (on the other side of the hall) and did so during the first week of the pain program. It was day three of the program, and because I had two conflicting appointments at the same time—one in group therapy and one for treatment—my decision was simple: I would go to the treatment appointment, which I ultimately did.

This was approximately two weeks after the first SGB I received. The second one was four weeks, and the third was six weeks, but then they became unsuccessful and I moved on to the next type of treatment. But because I didn't attend group therapy, I was approached by the nurse who scolded me for not attending group. Silly me thought that the two sides of the hall communicated with each other in the grander scale of the "comprehensive pain management program." I mean, how can you have a comprehensive program that doesn't include the treating physician for the pain diagnosis I was sent there for? Just didn't make any sense to me. I was so berated, that I walked away, running to a hotel near the airport, and calling a friend to pick me up and drive me home.

The next day, I made an appointment with my therapist and discussed the whole thing with him, including the part where "Doctor God" didn't believe my undercover story. The one thing "Doctor God" didn't know was that I was in therapy while I was undercover, so the therapist knew everything! It was his decision for me to quit the job in the end as it wasn't healthy for me emotionally. I'm not sure who called who, but after speaking to my BWC attorney, I was told that I needed to return to the pain program or it might look like I wasn't trying to help myself get better. After calling to return, I was told I had to wait three weeks before they had another opening, so I waited and then returned. This time, I explained to the nurse why I left, and that I would not apologize to anyone for leaving, and furthermore, wanted to be treated with respect this time around, not judgment. She thanked me for saying that and said that it showed I wanted to get better. This time when I met with "Doctor God" and the staff, they were all very cordial, not demeaning. It was night and day different! Maybe putting my foot down was the right thing to do and I should have done it in the beginning? I did find out that "Doctor God" and my therapist spoke on the phone, and that's why he suddenly believed my story. I am only grateful that I had a therapist that could back me up, but was angered that if I didn't, then I still wouldn't be believed.

I completed the program in three weeks and was glad to "graduate" from there and move on by April 1999. They informed all of us that we could come back to the group therapy any time we wanted, but I wasn't making any plans for sure! As the SGB's stopped being of benefit, my doctor talked about a trial for the spinal cord stimulator (SCS), which is an internal TENS unit that provides neural stimulation to decrease the pain. I had my trial in August of 1999, at the same time I was hosting a lady from Bosnia because of my work with the city. Naturally, nothing is easy for me, so the day after the trial SCS was placed, I had to return to the ER in Cleveland (since there was no one back home that knew about RSD) and as it happens, two of the Bosnian's friends drove me there that weekend. I found out that the stitches used to keep the "leads" in place broke and the leads were giving me electrical zaps. It was removed in the ER and I had a follow-up appointment with Doctor S.H., in the next two weeks where he decided the trial was a success and surgery for the real deal could be scheduled for November of that same year.

My parents took me to this surgery, which was outpatient at that time. On the way home, I remember being a pain in my own butt, literally! While the leads were placed in my spinal column, the battery pack was placed in my gluteus maximus.

I didn't realize how much muscle I had there until they took some of it out! No fun! I couldn't move without a great deal of pain.

I worked during all of the SGB's and trial SCS up until the final placement in November. And I thought I would be off for six weeks and then back to work. Well, that was the plan anyway. Once again, my body had other ideas about that. As you may be aware, any trauma can cause a diagnosis of RSD, including breaks, strains, sprains, bullet wounds, stabbings, and surgery. I just had a trial and final placement of an SCS, and I'm already feeling the spread of my RSD down into my right leg. Doctor S.H., prescribed Baclofen for my newly acquired spasticity (tremor-like twitching) and I knew a revision to the SCS is now required to add leads to the upper extremity.

Just for grins and giggles, I also started to experience a dramatic increase in seizures since the SCS placement. My neurologist had consulted with my pain doctor who told her that there was no correlation between the SCS and increased seizures, which she explained to me. But I knew there was no way it wasn't related I had gone from having one per year to now having 30 per day! And, though I'm not a doctor, it made sense that since a new electrical device was implanted, with leads up and down my epidural space, including in my neck, that combined with the brain (an abundance of electrical activity), it had to be the exact reason for these increased seizures. The neurologist would eventually come to the same conclusion years later, after another patient with an SCS also experienced seizures he never experienced before the SCS. Now I couldn't drive at all and had to rely on my then-boyfriend (later turned husband, then ex-husband) to drive me everywhere. I've lost my independence! I couldn't even hold my plate of food anymore because I was using Lofstrand crutches to ambulate (they are crutches that wrap around the upper arm for more support).

Sidebar now to discuss my personal history with marriage. I was divorced in 1993 from the father of my three children, way before the trauma that led to my diagnosis of RSD. But I was elated when I met my second husband post-RSD, who had said early in the dating stage, "I'm in love you, but I know I'm marrying you AND the RSD." The day before our backyard wedding in 2002, he told me, "I've never been so sure about anything in my entire life," when asked if he wanted to back out. Needless to say, he lied, because less than a year later, we were filing for a dissolution. To this day, I think it had everything to do with my RSD since I was in a wheelchair by this time.

Getting back to the history of my disease, I had three revision surgeries to my SCS in March of 2000, September of 2000, and April of 2001 before it was eventually removed in March of 2003, and since April of 2000, I had now reached systemic RSD. Difficulties with the leads, moving in the epidural space, making me jump off the table at the doctor's office, made it imperative for a fifth revision, but I told the doctor enough was enough already. Every surgery only caused the RSD to spread. It was in March of 2003 when an infusion pump (sufentanil and baclofen) was surgically placed, and the SCS was removed.

I did have a trial for the pump and was hospitalized during this time, and once again, the stitches that were supposed to hold it in place, broke and I was leaking epidural fluid so the trial was stopped, and the implant was deemed successful and scheduled for permanent placement. I later found out that my SCS data was used to make changes to the leads because mine, not only moved but broke and bent in other spots.

With no surprise, the seizures I was experiencing daily also ceased once the SCS was removed, confirming that it correlated.

Driving back and forth to Cleveland for pump refills began to take a toll on both my car lease in mileage and my sanity. I was offered a visiting nurse to perform the refills at my home, which continued through October of 2003 when I experienced a spinal headache an hour after a refill and had to visit a local ER for help. Naturally, I arrive at the ER and explain why I'm there only to be asked what I expected them to do since they didn't implant the pump. I pleaded with them that I just want the headache to go away! Up to this point, the number of pain meds I became allergic to had left me with few choices. I had allergies to Percocet, Stadol, Oxycodone, Ultracet, Demerol, Morphine, Vicodin, and Fentanyl, to name a few. So obviously I wasn't a run-of-the-mill opioid abuser looking for pain meds. I had called CCF, but the soonest they could see me was two weeks, and they instructed me to follow up with my local ER. By the time I saw the pain doc, it was too late for a blood patch, but the catheter was confirmed as out of position and another surgery was scheduled for revisions once again. During the wait, I thought more about another road down revision surgery, now for the pain pump, and contacted the doctor and requested that it simply be removed, which was approved and in November of 2003, the surgery was scheduled, and I was put on oral methadone.

During 2004, I had to seek a referral to a urologist because I was suffering from the inability to urinate either at all, or not emptying my bladder all the way. I was eventually diagnosed with "neurogenic bladder and sphincter diffuser" which meant I either had a Foley catheter in place, taped to my leg, or I would have to self-catheterized, neither of which I wanted to embrace. Needless to say, this had to be added to my allowed conditions in my BWC claim, which meant more hearings and more money to pay my attorney. I initially avoided this because I thought it would be too intrusive, and personal, for the supporting physician appointments I would have to make—on behalf of the BWC and my side. But in the end, I was convinced, and appreciative that I went this route. I was also driving back and forth to CCF for monthly methadone refill prescriptions which also took a toll on my leased vehicle and I barely drove it myself because I was using a wheelchair. At this point, both my legs and arms were weakened due to intense pain.

My pain doctor prescribed a lift for my vehicle to travel more independently with my wheelchair. In attempting to acquire this, my BWC managed care liaison, who was attending my doctor appointments with me, although we always had to drive independently of each other (something I never understood since BWC would reimburse me for gas and tolls to and from CCF), spoke with the mobility company service manager in my city.

Both of us were told the same thing: To accommodate me, I would need a van that was no older than 3-years.

That was pretty much the only requirement we were both told, so I bought a used van that was less than 3-years old. But the day I dropped it off to have the lift added, I was told that the van also needed to be an extended version, something they DEFINITELY NEVER told us! Now, I'm stuck with this van and no way to add a lift so I had NO independence.

The liaison was so upset she stated that she would NEVER use this company in the future with any other client. I had to wait two years before I could wrap the balance of this loan into the new car loan!

But I did eventually get approved for a modified van—the modifications were covered by BWC, but the van payment was my responsibility. I'm on my third modified van now—started with a 2005 Chevrolet Uplander, followed by a 2011 Honda Odyssey, and now a 2017 Chrysler Pacifica. I couldn't imagine my life without this vehicle and I highly recommend anyone with BWC claim allowances and systemic or lower extremity RSD to inquire into buying one for themselves.

After driving to CCF for methadone, and constantly listening for the "ah" from pharmacists filling my prescriptions (as if I'm a heroin addict now on methadone), I found a local pain doctor practice that didn't require a psychiatrist visit to be seen. In my view, I had already endured and graduated from that program and didn't have the desire to be told it's mandatory once again. I was successful, and even managed one small window of "remission" in the summer of 2008. I was able to ambulate just using my Lofstrand (forearm) crutches once again and it felt great! Unfortunately, it didn't last. The road out of remission was harsh and the pain seemed to be even worse than the first time around. I remember vividly the depression and even suicidal thoughts I had in 1999. Being a single mom of three small children meant that I was always supposed to be tough and not cry in front of my children. I felt less than a human being, much less their mother, and spent every night in tears crying into my pillow hoping they wouldn't hear me. I had to attend their sporting events, cheerleading games, and teacher conferences acting as if nothing was bothering me. I was even told by my ex's wife at these same sporting events (when attempting to discuss visitation issues with my ex) "Didn't you take your anti-depressants today?" I wanted to punch her lights out! But we were at church-related sporting events (CYO), so that option was out. Truth be told, my children are the only reason I kept from committing suicide.

In 2009, my current pain doctor had to refer me to another pain doctor because he could no longer control my pain and suggested I needed another trial for pain infusion pump therapy. This time, I had to see a psychotherapist and complete a computerized psychological profile to ensure my success. I was approved, but I was cautiously optimistic based on the first drug pump failure. Also, because the list of pain meds I was now allergic to had reached "nutville", I wondered what options I would have. As it turns out, I could take morphine in the small amounts I would be receiving through the infusion pump. Once again, a trial was performed, and naturally, the one big problem was my bladder was shutting down. I had to return to the doctor's office the next day and was sent to the ER from there to be catheterized. The nurse said I had the record for urine held then expended of 90cc. And from the container, believe me, it was a lot! This can be a side effect, and with my neurogenic bladder, I guess he should have forewarned me! I had the pump implanted in March of 2010 and it has been successful thus far.

I have had to have it increased from time to time, and eventually reached a plateau. After researching, I suggested adding bupivacaine and clonidine to the pump and surprisingly, my doctor agreed! I also had to be switched to Sufentanil, bupivacaine, and clonidine when the morphine couldn't be raised anymore because of my reaction to it. It seems to be working pretty well with increases about once a year.

The only problem I seem to be having lately is the PTM. I've had to call Medtronic (the manufacturer) twice in the last six months to replace the PTM's because they stopped communicating.

Two years later, I had urological testing and became a candidate for a bladder stimulator in June of 2012. Yep, just like it sounds. It's very much similar to the spinal cord stimulator in that it is an internal TENS unit to stimulate the nerves in my bladder to allow me to urinate without having to self-catheterize. My urologist called me the poster-girl for the bladder stimulator. Imagine THAT! I was doing great until they were wrong as far as when the battery would last. It suddenly stopped last August, about five years after it was implanted (no surprise to me), and I was scheduled for a revision in February of this year, 2019. Of course, it had to be BWC approved first, so the red tape took a while. I had the surgery, but within weeks, I had fluid seeping from the incision, which I couldn't see because it was in my left buttock! I don't know how many other people can kiss their own ass, but I can't! Two weeks post-op, I saw the nurse practitioner at the urologist office, who put some "butterflies" on the incision that was "super-glued" instead of stitches or staples, and I was put on antibiotics. Ten days later, I was still sleeping a lot and was told to visit the ER, which obtained a culture (negative) and bandaged again. Four weeks post-op when I visited the nurse practitioner again, I knew I would be having emergency surgery. I had my friend take a picture of my scar and saw it was so open (and red) that I could see the internal stitches, the lead and the device itself! What I didn't know is that I would have to have it removed, be hospitalized and released using a wound Vac, wait for this to clear up and heal, then have another surgery to implant it again, this time with an antibiotic pouch in the incision. I was told that I was nearly septic. Thank God I asked my friend to take a pic, and I called the on-call doctor the weekend before I had my return appointment! I'm just a few days away from the surgery to implant the bladder stimulator once again. This time, he will have to use the right buttock for battery placement. I'm not sure how that is going to go since I have scar tissue from the SCS battery pack in the same place.

The bladder stimulator nightmare was nearly a recreation of the pain pump battery replacement surgery! Just my luck! Most of my doctors now refer to me affectionately as "the One Percenter" --meaning, if 99% of the people have this happen to them, I don't. And conversely, if 99% are normal, I'm not! My pain doc scheduled me for a November 2016 battery replacement surgery. Two days after I saw them for the two weeks follow up, I ended up back at the ER (called the office as was referred to ER) because I was soaked through my shirt, my underwear, my sweats (it was winter folks) and I thought it was the meds themselves. What else could it be? Pain management and neurosurgery consulted with me and said it was lymphatic fluid, so they cleaned the incision and bandaged me up to see the pain doctor the next morning. He proceeded to apply "butterflies" sort of haphazardly.

The next day, I was back at the ER, and this time was told by neurosurgery that I would have to have emergency surgery (which was scheduled for my birthday) and possibly be hospitalized if it needed to be removed. Luckily, I wasn't hospitalized, and it didn't need to be removed (I couldn't see any part of the device). As if by a miracle, I had met the neurosurgeon who would also be doing another surgery in another two weeks—brain surgery!

Beginning on January 4, 2016, I had the worst medical luck of anyone I knew. I had been referred to an eye doctor due to increased blurriness only to find out I had sclerotic lenses (hardened lenses) due to prescribed steroid use. Who knew? Not me! I had to have cataract surgery on both eyes, two weeks apart.

As I looked around the day of surgery, with my oldest son there, I was the youngest person having cataract surgery. Everyone else was gray-haired and even white-haired. While I have a few gray hairs of my own, I'm pretty much still a blonde. I was seeing an orthodontist in Columbus, Ohio for a severe TMJ problem which required now the fifth surgery–arthroscopic surgery on the TMJ joint, which was outpatient and out of town in May of 2016, and a sixth surgical procedure for a jaw dislocation. I was also referred to an Ear-Nose-Throat (ENT) doctor who told me I had a deviated septum and sinus problems that needed surgical intervention right away. The local outpatient clinic was scheduled to do the surgery, but once again, the "One-Percenter" appeared. Just before I was taken back to surgery, I was told the anesthesiologists weren't comfortable doing the surgery, there because of my pain pump (they thought it was going to leak out somehow during the surgery... As IF!), so the IV was removed (I would have loved avoiding that for sure) and I was sent home to be scheduled later at the hospital.

Next, I was scheduled for a rotator cuff tear and SLAP tear surgery with the orthopedist. This was done literally at the end of the same week as the sinus/septum surgery--not same hospital though. Another outpatient surgery, I was sent home with an ice machine and a port for Carfentanyl IV medication. The night of the surgery, I felt like the port was leaking. They had sent me back to the ER the next day because I was in a GREAT deal of pain. And because of the RSD, I couldn't handle the blood pressure cuff going off every five minutes! I was sent up to surgery for a nerve block (on my shoulder called interscapular) where it leaves the arm limp and heavy...and for fun, you can use it to smack yourself in the face! That was the best they could do as there were no surgeons available to reinsert the IV port for the Carfentanyl. I had to come back to the pain management doctor the following day for yet another interscapular block, which is the last and only other pain management I had for the shoulder surgery. Shockingly to the surgeon, I was able to raise my arm totally at my first return visit ten days post-op. He told me no other patient has been able to do that, and I knew three other people who had the rotator cuff surgery done weeks before me that still couldn't move their arms. You go girl (I thought a lot then).

Before the year ended, I had the above-mentioned pump replacement surgery and had to have toenail removal surgery as well. My podiatrist calls it "diabetic feet" whatever that means, but basically, I guess it's neuropathic in origin. Because of my RSD, I can't have this done in the office and have to be seen as an outpatient in the hospital of course.

During the same time, I was struggling with awful occipital headaches (I called them "cough, headaches" because coughing, straining, lifting or bending over made them go off the charts) and had been scheduled for a brain MRI and CSF flow study. I was inpatient at one hospital for the headaches and had to be discharged so I could get the MRI at another hospital. The neurologist called an hour after the scan and told me I was being admitted back to the first hospital and the neurosurgeon came in the next day to tell me I needed brain surgery for "Chiari malformation," which means I had a brain hernia (cerebellum drops below brain stem).

This was the same neurosurgeon I had met for the emergency pain pump surgery now weeks before. And remarkably, the neurologist had referred me to this pain doctor when the occipital blocks stopped working, so I met him before I was referred to him by my first local RSD pain doctor for the pain pump surgery. The only thing they could give me for pain was Toradol and it wasn't working at all.

Somehow, they came up with Geodon (Ziprasidone) which worked GREAT! I found out that it's a psychotropic drug which is prescribed to schizophrenia patients. How they figured out it helped pain is beyond me.

I felt a huge relief after the surgery and told my surgeon, he was a miracle worker and thanked him so many times! It was just like the first successful SGB—a magic wand was waved over me and poof! The pain is gone! Remarkably, I received a call while I was recovering from this surgery in the hospital from the oral surgeon from Columbus, Ohio, who wanted to schedule the next TMJ surgery. I was getting a 3-D printed TMJ joint from California, and it finally came in. This was scheduled in two weeks, so I made sure it was okay from the neurosurgeon first, which he approved. I had to stay in the hospital for two days with this surgery. I remember vividly being in my hospital room post-op and having one heck of a whopping headache and nothing for the pain. I began to worry that the Chiari decompression surgery hadn't worked after all.

This was difficult because I had symptoms returning—primarily the occipital headaches. The doctor did consult with me before the first surgery informing me about the two choices I had before me and did so with great bedside manner. He acted like he was my friend, sat eye-to-eye with me, and explained everything so that I could understand, even in his heavy French accent (he was from Montreal, and I took French in high school). On one hand, a surgery that had minimal risk, but 20% of the patients needed a second surgery. And on the other hand, a surgery with more risk, and a 6% chance of needing a third surgery. My children wanted me to pick the latter because they knew me—I was that "One-Percenter!" But I couldn't pick the riskier surgery and opt for the first choice. Now I knew I needed the second, more risk surgery. He ordered another MRI-CSF flow study, which showed the CSF was restricted again and confirmed my suspicions. They scheduled the surgery and I repeated the hospital stay in ICU for the first two days, followed by another three days in the hospital. I was discharged to follow up with my array of doctors once again.

A mere month later, I was back in the hospital again with severe, debilitating headaches that felt like my head was going to explode. I had to wait in the lobby for my room to be ready and all the while trying to hide my tears because of the pain.

By the time my room was ready and they took my blood pressure, it was 160/83. I had brain surgery again, but this time to relieve the pressure with an intracranial shunt. I remained in ICU for three days until the pressure subsided and the decision was made to remove the shunt. Unfortunately for me, I missed my dad's 80th surprise birthday party!

My follow-up MRI and CSF flow study after the last surgery were marked by "artifact" and because they couldn't see it clearly, a myelogram was ordered by the new neurosurgeon (my great neurosurgeon had left the hospital).

At the next office visit, I was told I needed neck fusion surgery and that was scheduled before the end of the year. It was at this visit that I suggested that perhaps because of the RSD and the subsequent meds for everything, the result of which is constipation, maybe that was the real cause for my

Chiari (or brain hernia). He didn't give me any answers to confirm, but he didn't deny it either. Possible research paper topic? What I do know is that I had to make another appointment recently with the neurosurgeon because the "cough headaches" came back with a vengeance. The neurosurgeon asked me if I had any new films to show him. Really? How would I get those without them being ordered by a physician? I mean, I know what they're going to show...but I'm not a doctor. And of course, he had to order the MRI/CSF flow study which I was in a position to get done at this hospital this time because the bladder stimulator was out at the moment. I still had the pain pump, and always have to swing by the doctor's office for that to be looked at after an MRI because the MRI knocks the pump out! It always begins to work again...at least so far!

The follow-up appointment went horribly wrong—at least according to me. My cough was so bad that tears were streaming from my eyes, down my face to my mouth! The neurosurgeon, despite paying my $40 co-pay, decided I was "too sick" with "pneumonia" that he couldn't discuss the surgery with me, because basically, "I wouldn't be cleared for surgery in this state." He told me that I needed to come back in four weeks (appointment made for six weeks) and asked who I see for this cough. I replied, "I've called my pulmonologist for something for the cough, but they only called in antibiotics and more steroids." He said he would be calling the doctor and I provided the doctor's name and phone number. I know he never contacted him because I saw the pulmonologist myself a week later and asked if he heard from the neurosurgeon. He had not. And I had a chest X-ray which proved I didn't have pneumonia! This doctor wasn't happy with the other one because he said "How would he like it if I made diagnoses about your brain? He needs to stick to his specialty." In the meantime, I decided to get a second opinion on the matter which is scheduled for three days after the bladder stimulator surgery next week. I'll see the second opinion doctor before I talk to the first neurosurgeon. I'm hoping the second will have a better bedside manner!

This pretty much brings me back to the present—a few days away from the latest bladder stimulator surgery, and days away from information about more brain surgery! The only way I get through all this is by seeing my adorable twin granddaughters (who are 15- months at the time of writing). I babysit for them twice a week and sometimes even get to babysit overnight!

I've recently posted on social media that, the other thing better than being a mother is being a grandmother! I truly believe that. Yes, at the end of the day, I'm in pain. But I can sink into my bed and "veg" out watching TV, which usually means I fall asleep early, resting up until I get to watch them again. I do believe that helps me to avoid focusing on the pain EVERY MINUTE, but it doesn't distract me from the pain I feel when they grab my legs or arms. I haven't had the pleasure of being hugged by my children or other family members since I was diagnosed. I missed that and I mean A LOT! I could hug them, but just not BE hugged. The babies don't know any better, so they just cling on. It's comical to see them with me on the wheelchair. One step up on the foot stand and I have her turn around, so she faces away from me, while the other always wants to be picked up and eventually sits on my thigh.

I'm sure if I was looking at me, I would think it was funny and cute too! The other thing I found to be very helpful is music. Whether writing and playing original music or listening to Alexa play "top pop" on my Echo, it keeps me thinking about something other than my pain for the most part.

I even ask my pain doctors to let me take my cell phone and earbuds into procedure rooms. Surprisingly, they have allowed it for the most part. It's possible that I'm not the only one with the same requests?

I've had numerous thoracic and lumbar RFA's (radiofrequency ablations) with great results because of the many SCS surgeries, which has left me with thoracic facet joint disease (TFJD), according to my pain doctor.

Hundreds of nerve blocks and even more surgeries have allowed the RSD to spread to my entire body. However, I have to say that I like the pain pump over the SCS any day. I don't like the continuous buzzing that I feel with the stimulators. It's very hard to fall asleep with that every night. That's one thing I'm going to dread getting used to again with the bladder stimulator. I looked into ketamine infusion therapy, but there isn't any place locally that does it, so I continue to watch the support group chats to follow whether others have been successful with the different therapies. I firmly believe that support groups can help provide answers as well as support, especially to the newly diagnosed. I remember how scary that was for me and only wish Facebook was around back then. I started a support group for patients in NW Ohio, but quickly found out that most people would show up for answers to their questions, but then crawl back to the shadows, despite inviting speakers on various topics to address the group. It was disbanded after just one year due to low attendance, but most have found the RSD (now CRPS) support groups on Facebook. Our Facebook page is RSD/CRPS of Ohio.

Since RSD/CRPS is a central nervous system disease which affects the Sympathetic nervous system, I was well aware that it could cause problems for my muscles, soft tissue, skin, veins, bones, and other areas. I did not think about the side effects of all the medications I take. I know all about opioid addiction, but I never envisioned problems with my teeth. News flash--meds cause dry mouth, and I mean extreme dry mouth! All the Biotene in the world wouldn't help me and this issue led me down the road to tooth decay and ultimately, removal. Who knew? Not, me.

When my dentist referred me to a prosthodontist for a cavity, I knew something was wrong. It would have been nice, however, for the dentist to personally explain the reason for the referral, instead of having the receptionist call to inform me of the cancellation of the dentist appointment and referral.

I remember the tears flowing down my cheeks as I sat in the chair as the specialist, doctor dealing with dentures, explained my X-rays to me one red checkmark at a time. Each checkmark reflected another decayed tooth that needed to be pulled. Eventually, he checked every tooth in my mouth and explained I would also need implants, not just dentures because of my extreme dry mouth. One needs saliva for dentures to "sit" on the gums. I didn't have any, and therefore, my only option was to have implants--metal posts drilled into the jaw, usually three or four on the top and the bottom--to secure the dentures. I inquired about denture creams, as I thought that everyone uses because I've seen the ads on television. I was told again that it still requires saliva. The price tag for these implants: a whopping $50,000, and more tears flowed. How do people afford this? That's as much as half of a house! Naturally, the doctor had no advice for me.

Since I had been to see my oral surgeon during this time, I asked his advice for how I was going to pay for this, and he informed me that this was the "Cadillac of dentures." There were other options, including having him remove my teeth and insert the implants. And I would have opted for that if it wasn't for the fact that he was out of network for my insurance, so for every surgery, I had with him, the balance was not written off--I had to pay it. I did seek another opinion from my local oral surgeon who gave me another referral who was decidedly the most reasonable option at $2,200 for the dentures. The oral surgeon was the biggest cost for the removal and implants at just under $15,000, but this was not going to cause me to sell my house. I'm glad to report that the surgery went well and I am now a member of the denture wearing community. Unfortunately, for me, this didn't fall under my medical insurance, but my dental with a maximum yearly benefit of $1,300, it didn't cover much of the surgery cost. Add this to the list of body parts that this disease damages. No fun!

THE JOURNEY THAT CHANGED ME... MY CRPS STORY
By: Kira West

I thought I would start my story off by introducing myself. My name is Kira and I am from England. I am a 31-year old mother of two children and a wife of three years to my husband Jason. My story started three years ago when I was working as a caregiver for the elderly with dementia. I was settled in my job and loved it so much I found it so rewarding. I had been doing a shift at work just like any other day when I started experiencing discomfort in my left foot halfway through my shift, but I shrugged it off and put it down to being on my feet too much as I had done quite a few shifts prior. My mum came with my two children Mia and Oliver to meet me after my morning shift like they had done many times before, and we started to walk home as I had always done before, but this walk seemed different to the ones I had done in the past. We finally made it home, and I took my shoes off to rest my feet and hoped the discomfort I was feeling would ease as I rested, but it didn't. My mum and husband suggested that I take the following day off work and simply rest as they were worried, I had done too much and just needed to take it easy.

So, I took the following day off from work and tried to rest, but the discomfort had turned into pain and stiffness in my foot and I could barely move it. It had swollen up to double its size, and I couldn't even get my shoe on so we called the doctors and made an appointment for later that day to see if they could help at all. I went in and saw the doctor and they had diagnosed me with plantar fasciitis and sent me home. They had instructed me to rest it for two weeks and that it would soon ease, but what we didn't know is that was the worst thing I could have ever done. So, as the weeks passed the pain intensified and it was starting to affect my sleep and my day to day life. I hadn't been working in over two weeks because I couldn't bear weight on it and I wasn't even able to take my children to school or nursery as I couldn't get there so I was reliant on my friends and family to do this for me.

My husband took me back to the doctors, and they referred me to our local hospital for physiotherapy to see if that would help. So roughly two weeks went by and I was climbing the walls with pain. I couldn't sleep and was frustrated that I was unable to work and live my normal life taking the children to school and nursery, it all started to take its toll on me and my family, but we finally got an appointment to see a physio but unknowing to us, he would become a friend and a physio to me and my husband.

So, the day of my appointment arrived, my husband and I was anxious to see what would happen. We arrived and booked in and sat in a small waiting room wondering who would be seeing us. A gentleman by the name of D.P., came out and introduced himself to us as a physiotherapist (PT) and occupational therapist (O.T.). We went into a side room and started talking about symptoms and what I was experiencing, and he asked if it was possible to have a look and examine my foot.

I could not even bear him to touch it as it was so sore and painful. After a few minutes, his face changed and asked us to excuse him for a few moments as he needed to go and get another person for their opinion. So, off he went after a few minutes of my husband and I were sitting in a small room looking at each other wondering what on earth was going on? D.P., returned with a gentleman by the name of Doctor S.H. He examined my foot and was asking similar questions. After a while of talking and doing some examinations, both D.P., and Doctor S.H., explained that they thought I was suffering from a condition called complex regional pain syndrome (CRPS).

I had no idea what that was, but they explained a bit about the condition, and they said I needed to be booked into a pain management clinic and be seen there by himself, D.P., and his team. Meanwhile, to help with the pain and try to make me as comfortable as possible, they sent me around to the casting room, and they fitted me for a black medical boot to help brace and stabilize my foot and ankle, to try to make it more comfortable. They also gave me crutches as well to help me get around a little easier until my appointment comes through for the clinic. So, we went home and tried to make sense and digest what we had been told. We waited for a letter to come in the post for what would become the first of many pain management appointments.

Over the next few weeks, we received a letter and attended my first appointment. We got introduced to Doctor K.D., who would become my pain medication doctor and D.P., my P.T./O.T. that we had met at my first appointment. During the meeting, we had discussed in more detail what CRPS is and how it could affect my nerves.

There, I was prescribed oral morphine to help with my physical pain and try to help settle my nerve pain they prescribed me pregabalin which was to try to block my nerves. These appointments continued once a month with everyone involved and in between those I saw D.P., once a week to help with movement as my foot was getting stiffer and stiffer, and I was losing the ability to move it and control it. It was horrible I found it difficult to accept what was going on. I was constantly tired and felt so poorly all the time. I had gone from one very active person to someone who had to rely on everyone else to help me and do the things I should have been doing myself. As time went by my relationship with Doctor S.H., became difficult because I was unable to achieve what goals he had set out for me on a monthly basis and because of that things got hard between us communicating correctly etc.

After a month or so I was forced to use a wheelchair, unable to move my left foot and unable to visualize it. My brain had shut that part of my nerves off that controlled my limb and I was exhausted, upset, angry, frustrated and extremely confused to what was going on with my body.

I remember at one stage when I was seeing D.P., I asked him if they could amputate my foot as it was so painful and I saw it as a stupid hindrance as I couldn't do anything with it, but D.P. said that I would have been at the risk of developing phantom limb syndrome, and as such he didn't believe it was for the best. We tried mirror therapy many times and we were always talking about how I was feeling and how it was affecting my family and everything else. We had one more pain management appointment, and it all blew up between myself and Doctor S.H... He said I wasn't trying hard enough to get my foot moving and trying to regain control in my brain.

He said he wanted to try the Swiss method of (despite how much pain it would cause) forcibly manipulating my foot at an attempt to loosen my ankle at which I said no, as I knew in myself; I wouldn't be able to cope with it. After that, every session I was having in pain management I would leave in tears, and I was also tired, exhausted, in pain and deflated. I never thought this would ever end and didn't know what was going to happen over the next few months. My pain management kept messing and changing my medication as it wasn't easing the pain and I was a mess in my head and struggling to cope, which in turn meant everyone else was too. I had changed to a person that I didn't recognize in the mirror. Every time I looked, I looked more tired, more poorly and more unaware of what was going on around me everything went almost into a blur for months.

They started me on other medications and started talking to me about maybe going for counseling, as I was struggling so much. They booked me into a clinic to have an ultrasound on my vessels, etc., to see if they could see what was going on inside my leg and foot. With this procedure, they were going to numb my whole leg so that later that day when it had taken effect they were going to see if they could physically manipulate my foot to see what was causing it to be so stiff, whether it was because of the pain or something physical. I remember that day only too well. My husband and I arrived for my appointment with Doctor K.D., my pain doctor.

We were led into a room I had never been in before and I was told to lay down on a table on my side and was asked to lay very still. I made sure I couldn't see what was going on as I was so nervous, but Jason was there, and he held my hand and was watching what was going on. Doctor K.D., proceeded to insert a big needle into the back of my knee to numb my whole leg and to make it more comfortable to have the procedure carried out. I can't describe the pain I was in as she was doing it. It was awful, but I knew it had to be done. I remember holding onto Jason's hand so tight and I didn't want to let it go. After she had inserted the needle and scanned my leg, they sent us out to wait for an hour to let the anesthetic to take hold properly on my leg so that they could carry out the tests that they wanted to do without causing me an immense amount of pain.

So, we waited an hour and got called back in and Doctor S.H., was there and asked me if I could feel my leg, etc., before he touched it and as you would expect I was like yeah that's fine I can't feel anything but OMG man was I wrong. As he grabbed my foot and pulled it, I nearly passed out. The pain smacked me in the face like a freight train, and I scared everyone with my response. As you can gather, it wasn't very pleasant. It was apparent that the block hadn't worked the way it was meant to. They then started talking about a spinal cord stimulator (SCS) but they weren't too sure if that was the right move to do so before my next pain management they sent me for a lidocaine infusion and they said that should help me with the management of my pain alongside my other pain medication, but two weeks before my infusion, I had a few blood tests done to check my blood levels. They told me that I had to start taking calcium and vitamin D tablets as they said it showed I was deficient in both which wouldn't help when it came to my infusion.

So, fast-forward a few weeks I had my infusion which wasn't too bad, to be honest. It all went straight forward as it was meant to, which is good as you know with CRPS nothing is ever simple. So, Jason and I went to my next pain management appointment to speak with them about the SCS surgery. They decided not to proceed with the SCS surgery. They wanted to try a course of hydrotherapy once a week for six weeks, so we did. It drained me weekly as my foot went into over-drive. During my hydrotherapy sessions, my left foot became more painful as it couldn't regulate its temperature. While I was in the pool, my foot felt like it was being constantly scolded. When I would get out of the pool, it had the opposite effect on me. It felt like I had just shoved my painful foot into a freezer. In total, I had three courses of hydrotherapy treatments. Each treatment course was once a week for six weeks. This treatment was a no-win situation for me.

During this period, we were in discussions about what to do next to my foot and what to try next. The doctors finally decided at one of my pain management meetings that it looked like I had a contracture of my Achilles tendon and other tendons. They recommended that it needed to be released for me to progress. We understood the risks that it might make things worse by having an operation during a flare-up, but I had no choice if I ever wanted to make progress. Months had gone by and we hadn't gotten anywhere. So, let's fast-forward a few weeks. Finally, we had received a letter in the post to inform me of a date for my operation.

On the 11th of October 2017, which was in six weeks, and we had to start planning for the children's care and thinking of how to explain to them, what was going to happen. Mia had been worrying about what was going to happen. She's such a little worry wart bless her heart and the last thing I wanted was for her to be worried about things. Oliver was too young to understand what was happening, all he knew was Mummy had an "Ouchy" on her foot, and it needed fixing and the doctor was going to help Mummy.

So, as the weeks went by, I was getting more nervous and more anxious about what to expect. I had many operations before, but for some reason, this one felt so different, there was more on the line than the others I had done in the past.

So, a week before my operation, D.P., wanted to see me and find out how I was doing and if I had any questions. He was brilliant at supporting me and Jason. He answered any questions we had. So, it got to the night before and I was a nervous mess. I was worried about what to expect and what was going to happen when we got in there. I couldn't sleep, I was up most of the night worrying and thinking about things and worrying about the children as I would be away from them for a few days, and I didn't like the idea of that at all.

So, the morning of the operation came around, and we got taken to the hospital for 7:30 a.m., and they admitted me to the pre-op ward and I went through all the checks that were needed before they took me down for surgery. Jason was with me and helped me settle my nerves as I was feeling sick and scared as it had suddenly hit me properly for the first time what was going to happen, as I had spent weeks worrying about everything else and not fully concentrating on myself. So, the nurse came to get me and the walk down to theatre felt so long, I can't remember what the nurse and I spoke about, to be honest with you, it was all just a blur. We walked into the anesthetic room and they laid me down on the table and did the usual checks. I remember it was really cold in there and I was laying on the table shivering. I saw Doctor K.D. my pain doctor and she said "See you in there it will all be ok trust us" and then they injected me with a general anesthetic and that was it. I was asleep for three hours.

I woke up in recovery with a back-slab cast on and in huge amounts of pain and the first thought was oh my God, what have you done to me it's not supposed to be like this. The nurses came over and administered more pain relief. I also had what they call a popliteal catheter inserted behind my left knee to administer anesthetic to my leg to numb the pain and that was inserted during surgery. I was taken to the ward after I had come around properly and stopped feeling sick.

Jason was there waiting for me and I couldn't have been happier to see him. The day, after my operation the doctors came around and explained what they had done in surgery. So, they had lengthened my Achilles tendon and lengthened my tendons to my toes and they had shortened a lot and every time, they pulled my foot up during surgery my toes curled under. I don't remember much of the hospital stay, to be honest as I was so out of it on pain medication.

I was on a mixture of oral morphine, the popliteal catheter, tapentadol (Nucynta) and my pregabalin (Lyrica). I was allowed home after four days but was on strict bed rest for two weeks, which I needed as couldn't bare standing up even having to get up for simple things like going to the toilet was agony and resulted in me being sick because it was too much, but Jason and my mum were there every step of the way. The recovery at home was hard for the first few weeks, the pain I was experiencing was horrible on top of that, the medication was making me feel so poorly as I was on a high dose of quick-release tapentadol as I couldn't get my pain under control.

I was in my back-slab cast to allow for swelling etc, and after two weeks I went for my first cast change to a normal cast. That should have been a straightforward procedure, but as they took the back-slab cast off to change it to the other one. My foot dropped and wouldn't stay in the correct position so instead of only having two casts for the next eight weeks I had to go back in every week and have it changed to adjust the angle of my foot to gradually bring it up to where it needed to be. That in itself was so painful as it all depended on where they cut the cast to remove it.

So, I finally came out my casts after 10-weeks of back-slab casts and normal casts and they transferred me into an air-boot which was easier as I could remove it to have a bath and help soak my foot as I couldn't stand having a shower on it as the pressure of the water made me cry and be sick. Jason had to help me the few first times I had a bath as I had to have tape on my toes to help splint them and avoid them contracting again. We had to have my foot soaking in the bath to help remove it all and I'm not going to lie it was agony. My husband sat with me in the bathroom carefully removing the tape off of my toes and it took over an hour of me sitting in the bath with tears streaming down my face. After the removal of the tape, I was exhausted emotionally and mentally. I felt very detached from my foot I kept looking at it that night and didn't really recognize what was there. It looked distorted and not what I remembered. It had a big incision and stitches that weren't there before. I had struggled for over a year to recognize my left foot this is all part of this horrible disease it felt like my brain had detached itself almost.

As weeks went by every day, I would sit and look at it with no emotion towards my limb apart from hate. The pain was awful, it never seemed to ease. I couldn't control the movement at all. I struggled to connect my brain with my limb I would sit for hours staring at it, willing it to move and wondered if I would ever be able to regain control of this lifeless limb that hung from my left leg. I had gone into muscle atrophy in my whole leg because of it. What was, someone's abnormal had become my normal life and it was scary and upsetting.

My family rallied around and tried to help me with the " Touch it, love it, feel it" motto that we had adopted during my journey. But I was struggling as every time I looked at it, it hurt me inside. I could see how it was affecting the children and how it had impacted on my family.

I hit a dark patch within myself and for a short while, I wasn't sure how I was going to make progress if any. It took weeks for me to see any way forward and to see how we could make the best of what had happened. Fast-forward a month and I had started looking at my foot more and accepting its new look. I was in my space boot for quite a few months as it was needed to help support my lifeless foot and to enable it to start healing from the inside out.

We gradually started to move my foot manually as I still couldn't control it from my brain.

As the weeks went on, it got easier and easier and slowly, I started to twitch my toes, which were a huge milestone for me as I hadn't been able to do that for so long. It took a lot of tears and angry outbursts due to frustration, but I started making slow progress at home with movement, etc. I received an appointment in the post (mail) to attend a pain management clinic the following month, which I was nervous about going as I didn't know what to expect as it was the first time, I had seen them since before my operation.

So, a month had gone by and my husband and I attended my appointment, and we all sat and discussed everything and where to go from here. At my appointment, I was given another black support boot to replace my air boot, when I was ready and to make it more comfortable and to ease the weight on my leg as anyone that has had an air boot knows they are quite heavy, cumbersome and uncomfortable.

My husband and I worked so hard at home with my recovery and rehabilitation. I finally made it into my black boot a few weeks later and that's when the hard work started. I was given photocopies of left feet and right feet to try and trigger my brain to recognize the difference between the two as I couldn't tell them apart which was so frustrating. People think this disease just affects the limb, but it doesn't, it affects everything and it was scary to think it had affected my brain and I hadn't realized how badly.

71

I had so much support over the next few months to get things moving and get me further on the road to recovery and to find our new normal again.

As months went by, I slowly regained some control over my foot and started moving it more and more as the weeks, and months went by. I was back and forth every week to see my physio and he helped me to try and understand the new journey I was on and to help me to focus on what we were aiming for at the end.

It took tears, a huge amount of determination and a lot of defeated days to make progress but that's only normal. Fast-forward a few months and I was finally able to put my foot on the floor and not cry and freak out because of the pain. I had many pain management appointments and many talks and many more physio sessions, but I finally managed to put a shoe on which was just amazing. I hadn't worn matching footwear for over two years. This was a huge milestone in our journey. I was still using crutches to help support myself, but I started to slowly walk very short distances and that grew and grew over time. The pain never leaves, but my tolerance level has increased. I remember I had one pain management clinic appointment and for the first time in my whole journey, I actually hobbled/walked into my appointment. I had never done that before.

By the next month, I went to what I didn't know at the time would be my final pain management clinic appointment. My husband and I showed up, we wondered what would be in store for us and what would be said, but as I walked in, I was greeted with smiles and them clapping for me as I walked in bold and steady on both my feet. They said they were so proud of my journey and how I had beaten the demons that had been with me only years before.

We sat and chatted and I looked at Doctor S.H., Doctor K.D., and D.P., and they had huge smiles on their faces and they said in unison that I was to be discharged from the pain clinic as a CRPS Hero and if I needed them, I could always go back. I remember that feeling of just pure self-accomplishments and that I had beaten this disease, and it hadn't beaten me.

My husband and I shook their hands and thanked them for everything and for the last time walked out of the clinic doors, but this time without tears in our eyes just smiles on our faces. We sat out in the front of the hospital to take a few minutes to let it all sink in that we had done it. We called everyone and told them the amazing news that I had been discharged and that it was for the first time just us as a family, no more doctors' appointments, no more surgeries, and more tears and the feeling of being defeated. It's been just over a year and things are continuing to develop and progress in the right direction. I can walk unaided; I can take my children to school and not rely on anyone else to do it for me and I finally feel like I am a mum again. I still have CRPS in my foot and I am still on opiate pain meds and still on nerve blockers to aid me in my day to day life, but you know what, that is such a small price to pay. Yes, I walk a little differently than I did before my journey and I still can't run like before, but I don't care. I have both my feet working and I have a new kind of normal again. I just feel incredibly lucky. I never knew how much I took for granted before all this, but I know now how important the little things are and how you should celebrate every milestone big or small as nothing is insignificant with this disease.

I know I will always have this disease in my life and my family's life's and I know it will always be waiting to give us another fight, but we have got this far once and we know we can do it again. I just wanted to finish my story by saying that nothing is ever impossible. I accomplished the impossible in my journey and you can too!! OWN your CRPS don't let CRPS own YOU!! Thank you so much for reading my story and believe nothing is ever impossible no matter what this disease throws you. Create your own kind of normal!!!

RSD – TESTIMONY
By: Nadège Gassend

I would like to introduce myself. My name is Nadège, I am 25-years-old and I am French. Since I was a child, I always had a problem with my balance. So, I always had fallen with injuries. In total, I had sprained my left foot eleven times. Following that, at the age of 12, I had surgery on my left foot to fuse my foot with screws. Fifteen days after my surgery they removed the plaster cast, Once, again, I had a balance problem. I had fallen again and I broke my fibula. So, once again, I was placed into another plaster cast for one month.

Gradually, I started to develop unbearable pain in my left foot (I had burning pain, electric discharges, feelings of pins and needles, feeling of soreness, anesthesia, stab wounds, feelings of vice, sharp pains, etc...). My foot changed (I developed a deformity and skin color change). It also became swollen. I was finally diagnosed with reflex sympathetic dystrophy (RSD) or as they call it now complex regional pain syndrome (CRPS).

The surgeon who followed my case since my surgery wanted to send me to a pain center. But my family doctor who followed since I was a child, did not want me to go to the pain center. In, 2007, I had a surgery to remove the screw that I had in the foot. Once again, my surgeon insisted that I go to the pain center.

I finally went to see the pain specialist. He wanted to perform a nerve block on me. He said that these blocks were normally done six months after the diagnosis of the RSD. The nerve blocks did not work on me. The doctor asked the hospital for authorization to give me another nerve block, but the hospital rejected his request because I was so young. So, the doctor decided to treat me with a few different medications like Tramadol,

Neurontin, Lyrica, etc... but I was intolerant. Following the therapeutic failures. He decided to send me to another pain doctor to perform mesotherapy (a procedure in which multiple tiny injections of medications are delivered into the mesodermal layer of tissue under the skin). I did this treatment for one to two years, but I was still having more pain. Subsequently, I learned that this doctor injected me with a placebo. Which explains why I had more pain.

My family doctor who followed my care, wanted me to stop seeing this pain doctor. He decided to put me on Fentanyl. Except that, he increased the doses of Fentanyl so fast. I was feeling so badly from the increased dose. He decided to stop the treatment suddenly overnight. After that, in 2013, I had a cerebrovascular accident. Next, I was put on morphine (my current doctor who followed my care wanted me to stop the morphine). Meanwhile, I did not stop the medication because of the falls that I was having. I had a lot of injuries which increased the RSD. I saw a neurologist who diagnosed me with Dystonia, but he did not want to follow my case because I was too young (I was 19-years old).

Afterwards, I decided to contact the first pain doctor again. He decided to see me again, in May of 2014, to do a peripheral nerve block. But he stopped everything because this block had a beneficial result, only to the color of my foot. This block did not have a beneficial effect on my pain. So, the doctor decided to remove the peripheral nerve block.

After that, in June 2014, the dystonia declined and the surgeon who has followed me since I was 12-years old, had to perform a surgery to extend the Achilles tendon. But, when he pulled the plaster cast off, the foot fell downwards again because of the dystonia. So, my RSD was put aside so we could focus on the dystonia for the next five years.

However, no neurologist wanted to take charge of my case because I did not come in one box. My situation started to deteriorate. I do have partial epilepsy, and the crisis of dystonia every day. All the neurologists that I saw refused to take my case on, some of them said that I pretended to have all the symptoms.

There were a lot of medical mistakes that I found recently. A neurologist who confirmed the presence of RSD, partial epilepsy and Dopa-responsive dystonia (Segawa disease). This neurologist hospitalized me to find a treatment. She also wanted to work with my pain doctor who follows me to find a pain killer to help my RSD pain. I am intolerant to some pain killer and others pain killers can accentuate epilepsy. The doctor recommended that I should try using a capsaicin ointment. I used it for one month. Concurrently, for one year, I use meditation in conscience and hypnosis as alternative treatments for my pain.

I have suffered from RSD for more than 13-years. It has impacted my personal life because I missed a lot of family events. I was put aside from a lot of people at school, I did not have friends because of that. I also enormously suffered from solitude, I lacked other-confidence because I suffered physically. I also enormously lacked self-confidence too, because people hurt me a lot because I am unwell. People also have abused me because of my confidence. Nevertheless, I now concentrate on my studies, which has given me a goal to look forward to. I am working on my receiving my Ph. D in Law, so I can help the highest number of people who have problems.

Nadège Gassend

"SEARCHING FOR HELP": HANNAH'S CRPS STORY

By: Janet

My daughter Hannah was an active, healthy eight-year-old child. All that changed on August 25, 2005. She was at soccer practice. It was raining. She rolled her left ankle into a shallow hole in the field. I had suffered numerous ankle sprains as a child. I broke my ankle twice while walking and had dislocated my kneecap twice. I thought it was simply a sprain. We took her to a Podiatrist that our Pediatrician recommended. They took X-rays. Nothing was broken, so they tightly wrapped it in a soft cast. She was given crutches and told to stay off it for two or three weeks. When we returned to this podiatrist, and he unwrapped the ankle, she screamed in pain. She was unable to bear weight or even have it touched. She couldn't move it and it became locked in a fixed position with her toes pointed up. The doctor could not understand why she was still in pain, or why she was acting this way. We were told to take her to a psychologist. He recommended a behavioral therapist. I knew she was not making this up. She went from being a happy, smart athlete to a scared, depressed child. The behavioral therapist was extremely aggressive, both physically and emotionally. It was abusive. After several months, I fired her.

Meanwhile, about two months after her injury, Hannah complained of severe stomach pain and did not want to eat. This was totally out of character, she LOVED food. We had no idea these two problems were related. We took her to Arnold Palmer Hospital in Orlando, FL. They did an endoscopy and a colonoscopy, which looked normal. They told us she was making up the pain. I again knew this was not true. She continued to lose weight and tell us her foot and now whole leg and stomach were in severe and constant pain. I searched and searched for answers. There was little information about complex regional pain syndrome (CRPS) back then. I stayed up many nights looking on the internet. She was terrified of doctors by this point because of how she was not believed or respected.

A year went by and she was still in excruciating pain. Her little leg was purple. She had lost about 30 pounds. The DCF was called. It was a nightmare for all of us. I don't know why, but I decided to try one more doctor. I did not even tell her where we were going. He was a pediatric orthopedic doctor. His name was Doctor L.R., He heard her symptoms and within minutes, he took me out of the room. He told me she had reflex sympathetic dystrophy (RSD). I cried because we finally had an answer. She was validated and believed. A weight was lifted off our shoulders. It WAS REAL! He explained that he could not treat it. We had to find a Pediatric Neurologist. I found Doctor M.H., from Palm Bay, FL. There was hope! He was very kind and compassionate. He did not treat children but knew all about RSD and had many adult patients with it.

Again, we were hitting a wall. Our pediatrician knew a pain management doctor who was willing to see her. At first, he was kind, he told us she had to have a sympathetic nerve block. He said that she would be admitted to the hospital and the block would be left in place like an epidural for five days.

She was terrified. This doctor, Doctor D., was not a pediatric doctor. He was willing to try and we were grateful for that. After about two or three days, it was not working at all. Her pain was the same. The medication was giving her hives and extreme itching. I told him we were going to leave and thanked him for trying. He screamed at me and told me I was not a good mother. I was devastated. His method did not work, so he blamed me and Hannah.

I would soon realize many doctors and healthcare professionals would do this to us, instead of trying something else, or considering that all patients are different.

All patients do not respond to treatments the same way. She was blamed for not improving. It was horrible. We tried physical therapy at several places. They did not know what RSD was and wanted to grab her leg and bully her into submission. It only made her more fearful and less compliant. We had a close friend who was a doctor. He thought we should take her to Shand's Hospital in Gainesville Florida. It is a teaching hospital with a great reputation. They thought it was psychological, even though she had a diagnosis. He referred us to an expert in RSD, Doctor A.T., She was kind and knowledgeable. She put Hannah on a high dose of Methadone. That was a huge mistake. She became bedridden. She was extremely frail and small. She could not do anything.

We did more research and decided to take her to Doctor D.R., in Corpus Christi, Texas. He had invented the VECTTOR Therapy System that helped RSD patients walk again. I was so hopeful. She could not fly, so I drove her there from Florida. We bought his machine. I think it was $6,000.00. This device was not covered by our insurance. He was very kind and knew so much about RSD. He had patients from all over the U.S and other countries. We stayed for about six weeks. Unfortunately, this treatment spread her RSD to her hands. They locked in fists with dystonia. It did help her stomach pain for about a week.

We had to find another way to help her. We researched again. There were pediatric pain programs for RSD in Boston, Cleveland, and a few other places. We decided on Cleveland because an expert on RSD Doctor M.S.H., practiced there. We drove her up there and he wanted to do a spinal cord stimulator trial. He made her do it with no anesthesia. It was horrible. The stimulator did not help at all. He made us put her in the pain program. It was supposed to be for three weeks. She was so bad by then, she stayed for months. It was brutal physical and occupational therapy, aqua therapy and basically coping with the pain. The program helped other kids who were not as severe as her. Her RSD had spread full body. She also had dysautonomia, gastroparesis, and later we would learn she had Ehlers Danlos Syndrome (EDS) which is a connective tissue disorder that is genetic. I had it too. Many CRPS patients have these comorbidities. It took about six more years for her to be diagnosed with EDS, postural orthostatic tachycardia syndrome (POTS), gastroparesis and dystonia. Our experience at the Cleveland Clinic was not good. They again blamed her for not improving in their " One size fits all" pain program.

We decided to take her to the new Nemours Children's Hospital in Orlando, FL. We told them her story. The pain management doctor, Doctor S., was sympathetic and appalled at how she had been treated. She promised to help Hannah. We were also referred to Doctor R.B., in Jacksonville Florida. He did a stellate ganglion nerve block and sent her to Brooks Rehabilitation Hospital. She stayed there for eight weeks. It made her worse again. Her stomach got worse too when they prescribed the wrong medications. So, she underwent a lot of tests at Nemours. She was finally diagnosed with gastroparesis and POTS. They treated her for a year, they did many procedures, such as Botox injections, casting and physical therapy. Once again, when she did not improve. They blamed her and said it was a conversion disorder.

Even after they had diagnosed her with these disorders and treated her for them. We were discharged from their care with no help.

We went back to Shand's Hospital and were treated horribly. We went to our local ER and they had no idea what she had or how to treat her. We then took Hannah to see Doctor A.K., in Tampa, FL. He did six Ketamine infusions for her. He was knowledgeable, but the infusions did not help her CRPS pain. They did help her stomach pain for a few days.

After 10-years, we finally found respect from a doctor. We went to Doctor A.H., in Clearwater, FL. He is THE MOST compassionate, knowledgeable and kindest doctor period. He promised he would help her. He knows all patients are different and treats them as individuals. He does NOT have a "one size fits all" approach. He treated her with high dose Ketamine infusions along with physical therapy.

We also found Doctor O.F., in Jacksonville, Florida. He was also appalled at all she had been through. He referred us to Doctor G., a Neurosurgeon in Jacksonville, FL. As a last resort, she got an intrathecal pain pump in 2015. Her GI system had completely stopped functioning by this time, She, had to get a central line put in. She was on TPN (total parenteral nutrition). She was hospitalized for a pulmonary embolism. She had sepsis twice from her central line.

She kept fighting. She never gave up. She fought for 10-years and 4-months. Finally, on December 27, 2015, she lost her battle at the age of 19. She always tried to help others with her disorders. She had many friends across the country.

She participated in the Documentary Film " Trial by Fire" which is about CRPS. She never got to see it. Her hope was to educate and spread awareness. Early diagnosis and treatment are the keys with CRPS. NO ONE, especially a child should ever have to go through this.

A JOURNEY FROM DESPAIR TO HOPE
By: I.D.R.

In August 2017, our 17-year-old son broke his leg at football practice the summer before his senior year. The X-ray showed a broken fibula in two places and one of the pieces of bone was pinching the Peroneal nerve. The orthopedic surgeon was concerned about foot drop because of possible damage caused to the perennial nerve. He warned us that foot drop might still be present even after surgery to repair the fibula. Foot drop would require our son to wear a brace on his ankle for the rest of his life. Little did we know then that "foot drop" would have been way better than the complex regional pain syndrome (CRPS) he ended up with.

Immediately after the surgery, his pain spiked more than he had in the four days waiting for surgery. Our son Austin was in excruciating pain. The hospital discharged Austin with a cryo-ice machine to help with the swelling and a prescription for pain killers which are normal for a fibula repair like the one that Austin had done. Four days after surgery, the surgeon reached out to us to check in on Austin and how he was doing. We told him that he had been in constant pain and could not get off the couch without assistance and that the foot was discolored (pink). The surgeon instructed us to bring him into his office. He diagnosed the color change from the calf down to his toes and touched, his foot lightly and then applied a little pressure on the foot's affected area. In both instances that the foot was touched the response was the same. The pain was excruciating for our son. The surgeon informed us that Austin most likely had reflex sympathetic dystrophy (RSD) – another term for CRPS. Austin could not put any weight on his leg. He was bedridden (actually couch ridden). He required help for everything, getting to the restroom, bathing, etc. The surgeon made a referral for Austin to see a Pain Specialist.

Twenty days after surgery in September 2017, we visited the pain specialist. We were so excited to learn this doctor studied CRPS at Harvard.

We could not believe in our small town we were able to find someone with knowledge about this disorder. The doctor explained how painful CRPS is and compared it to the pain an amputee feels. He planned out six sympathetic lumbar nerve blocks over the next several weeks. Each block provided a few hours of relief and at this point, we were grateful for every minute of relief. We had him doing physical therapy three times a week, and we scheduled those close to the nerve blocks, so he would have less pain and more mobility. The doctor also started Austin on gabapentin. The dosages were increased to the max of 1800 mg a day. The pills helped with some of the electric shocks he would get however the side effects were less desirable. Austin was "foggy," unable to answer questions or remember simple things. He was still unable to put weight on his leg and so he was confined to the couch. He could not even have the ceiling fan on because he could feel the pulse of the fan blades blowing air on his foot. The airwaves hitting his foot would cause throbbing pain. We made a box so he could put his foot inside to keep the airwaves from causing him any additional discomfort. His leg was purple and swollen. The hair on his leg would hurt him. A sheet touching his skin was too painful. We made a box over his leg so he could have a sheet on his body at night.

He could only move around with the help of crutches. His skin temperature was hot, he would be sweating even if the temperature was cold. Sometimes just his leg, other times his whole body.

After the six lumbar blocks were completed, the pain doctor (the "Harvard CRPS specialist") wanted to take a "wait and see" approach to our son's care. We tried to follow his advice, but our son was in so much pain. We began to research alternative treatments for CRPS.

We asked the doctor about ketamine infusions. He was completely against it. We felt we now had to put our son's care in our own hands, as we could not see him in this pain.

It was difficult to find medical professionals truly familiar with CRPS. Although the pain specialist had extensively studied CRPS, he was only willing to do the six blocks, medicate our son with pain killers and make a referral for physical therapy. We were so disappointed and had a hard time finding doctors, but we eventually found great doctors. We called numerous Neurologists but no luck. Little did we expect to have such a hard time finding a specialist however CRPS is rare. We ended up finding help where we did not expect. It was a doctor specializing in regenerative treatments and chiropractic care surprisingly offered the most help and hope.

Against the pain doctor's advice, we scheduled our son for two weeks of ketamine infusions. The infusions were all-day outpatient. Our son slept through most of the infusions and we were grateful he could sleep. The dosages were increased, and his pain diminished from a 10 to a 7-6 on the first day of treatment. That was the first time in months that he was able to sleep in his bed. As the ketamine infusions continued, and the dosage increased, the pain kept dropping. We were able to get it down to a 5-4 on the pain scale. The Ketamine infusions treatments were not covered by insurance and were expensive. As parents, we did everything we could, using our savings and taking out a hardship withdrawal from our retirement account to pay for all the treatments that we did to keep our son from being in the pain that he was in. Eventually, after many appeals, our medical insurance reimbursed us for part of the Ketamine infusions. If the insurance company denies treatment, do your research and submit appeals. I resubmitted several times and eventually, they were approved.

Austin continued to do physical therapy and aqua therapy. The aquatic therapy pool was an hour away. We would drive there three times a week.

It was the only time we could see our son "walk" again without assistance while in the water. I broke down in tears every time. These therapies were giving him some more movement, but he was in a lot of pain. I did a lot of research and tried acupuncture for two months as well. Austin did not feel much of a difference. I continued to search for more treatment options. My husband and I felt we were racing against a clock because the best chance of remission from CRPS is within the first six months to a year. At this point, we were almost five months in, and he was still unable to walk without crutches. Our search led us to stem cell.

We found facilities that were in Florida, but they were expensive. Luckily, I came across a physician locally who had started a new functional and regenerative practice. I contacted this doctor, and he had been a pain doctor for some time and was tired of masking people's pain.

He was familiar with CRPS but asked us to wait until he could learn more before treating our son. It just so happens he was set to attend a seminar for physicians treating CRPS with stem cell. I could not believe the luck and so we waited.

I will mention this doctor's name because I believe he was a Godsend to our family. His name is Doctor Jonathan Tait and his practice is in Oro Valley, AZ. He ended up doing two procedures on Austin a few months apart (November 2017 and February 2018). Both procedures were stem cell transplants (from Austin's hip) and Platelet Rich Plasma (PRP). Since Austin's CRPS was a result of a major nerve injury, we felt targeting the site of his nerve injury with stem cells could repair some of the damage. Doctor Tait injected the stem cells into the myelin sheath near the injury site. Before these treatments, Austin's entire foot was the majority of where he felt his pain. He had numbness and shocks in his calf near the injury site.

After the procedures, Austin's pain decreased and the numbness and shocks were less. It was a turning point. The pain doctor was against this procedure as well and probably many people with CRPS would be afraid to have needles injecting into their area of pain however it was a risk Austin was willing to take.

Austin felt the stem cells could not damage him, only heal him. He was still in a lot of pain and discomfort and he felt frustrated with his inability to walk and live his life. After each stem cell and PRP, Austin reported feeling a difference, a reduction in pain and less numbness and shocks. His rehab was moving in the right direction. Doctor Tait recommended Hyperbaric Oxygen Treatment to help with stem cell growth. I had read this treatment had been helpful for some people with CRPS. There was a clinic offering HBOT treatment about an hour away. This was also an expensive treatment not covered by insurance. Within three HBOT treatments in late October 2017, Austin's pink-purple leg began to look normal. After seven treatments, both of his legs were the same color and size (not swollen).

He completed many treatments (45) at the clinic, however to cut down on costs, we purchased a home HBOT. He uses the home HBOT daily and finds it very helpful.

Doctor Tait also wanted Austin to not be reliant on pain pills or gabapentin. It was this physician who helped us come up with a plan to wean Austin off these drugs. Doctor Tait also wanted Austin to change the way he ate. We had read before how certain foods (sugar, pork, etc.) can cause more nerve pain and so we figured let's do this plan. The doctor had him tested for food allergies and sensitivities and put him on a strict plan. Again, the pain was reduced and other symptoms he had been having were also reduced. Austin had a lot of digestive issues after starting the gabapentin. The diet helped with this as well.

Still, our son was mostly homebound and only able to go to school for a few hours a day. This was his senior year. He had been a popular kid with lots of friends. He was on the football team and his hopes for an athletic scholarship were out the door. He was unsure he would even be able to complete the 12th grade or graduate?

Socially, it was very difficult. Many friends came by when he had initially broken his leg. When he was diagnosed with CRPS, friends seemed to dwindle. People simply don't understand the disorder and the level of pain. Eventually, only a few friends checked in and visited.

It broke our hearts to see how a happy 18-year-old boy with his whole life ahead of him was now depressed and in pain, and alone except for his family. There were many nights he cried and shouted: "why?" As parents, we felt the same "why?" We feared for him; we were afraid he was going to commit suicide. We put him in counseling, even though he did not want to go.

So now he's seven months into CRPS (March 2018), and we kept searching for a cure. Now, I know there is no cure, but I prayed every day for one, I still do. I had seen on the internet some had success with Calmare. We showed the testimonials from Doctor Michael Cooney's website to Austin. It gave him hope. He was still weaning off the gabapentin, but this gave him the motivation to wean off since you cannot be on nerve medications for Calmare treatment. We set up flights and hotels for a few months away to go to New Jersey for Doctor Cooney's Calmare treatment. We prayed this idea would be the cure or at least the path to remission. Our son graduated high school.

We had dreamed of him walking across the stage to get his diploma, walking without a thought of pain but that was not the case. He walked with a cane and he had pain, but we were so proud of everything he had overcome.

June could not come sooner. The flight was so difficult for him; the air pressure causes someone with CRPS more pain. He was still using a walker

87

or crutches to get around. He was unable to wear shoes. The only shoes he could wear on his CRPS foot was a diabetic slipper, which has Velcro straps allowing it to have more room. He still had to apply either a ketamine cream or a lidocaine patch to help numb the top of his foot. Wearing a regular sock was hard as well, but he could tolerate wearing a fuzzy sock on his foot. We arrived and met Doctor Cooney the next day. This man was another angel in our son's life.

Doctor Cooney explained scrambler therapy to us. I would have never thought something like this could help anyone but when you are desperate you are willing to try it all. As a family, we were desperate; we deeply wanted our son to live without this pain and to be able to walk! The treatment was painless. Other than the doctor touching his foot, which any touch was uncomfortable, the electrodes do not hurt. They emit a painless signal.

In the first few days, there was not much decrease in his pain. However, Austin slept a long time, which was unusual. The doctor was determined to help Austin and would change up the placement of the electrodes daily. Finally, a few days later, Austin reported feeling less pain and being able to touch his foot. We located an HBOT clinic in the New Jersey area, and he continued with this as well. After a week with continued improvement, we asked the doctor if we could double up on treatments, he agreed as Austin was showing signs of improvements.

When Austin completed the Calmare treatment in mid-June 2018, he could wear shoes and did not need a walker or the ketamine cream or lidocaine patches on his foot. He could even touch his foot. It was for us, a miracle! For the next month, per Doctor Cooney's instructions, no physical therapy, just REST.

This was scary advice to follow as we were afraid, he would regress, however, we had Austin follow the advice. He was in almost no pain. He was at a level 2 to 4. He could walk unassisted!

He was slow, but he was walking. After a month of rest, he started walking on a treadmill daily and increased his level of activity. He also started going to college two days a week, so that also helped to get him walking and back to a normal routine.

After a few months, some pain started to return. As per Doctor Cooney sometimes a Calmare booster is needed to settle the affected nerves back to their normal state. Luckily for us, we found Doctor Wade in Glendale, Arizona only two hours away.

We took him in for a Calmare booster, three treatments. Austin's pain was now down to a 1 to 3. The last Calmare booster was over a year ago in August of 2018. I am happy to report that Austin is in remission, not cured but not in pain. He worked up to wearing various shoes and he was able to do this by using a tub of rice and immersing his feet in the tub for 10 to 30 minutes a day for desensitization. He continued on the treadmill and was in such great shape he went snowboarding various times last winter.

Snowboarding was his goal and it was tough to get there. The boots are painful, and he knew he had to get used to the shoes and improve his stamina and balance. He worked hard every day using snowboarding as a goal, and his hard work paid off. Austin's rehab was almost four hours a day. It included two hours HBOT (home chamber) and two hours on the treadmill, exercise bike, and weights. He also did the rice desensitization daily until he felt he did not need it. In, December 2018, Austin went snowboarding, incredible recovery from having been bedridden the year before and unable to walk!

CRPS remission is not like a cancer remission. There are still occasional shocks and a lot of stiffness, especially in the morning. Austin gets up an hour earlier and sometimes uses a cane until he does not feel stiff. He can finally sleep in his bed with sheets, but he wears a fuzzy sock on his CRPS foot because though he does not feel pain, the sensation of sheets feels awkward. Weather also impacts him. Cold can cause more joint stiffness.

Every CRPS case is different and what works for one person may not work for another. This story is what helped my son. There are things I wish we would have known from the beginning and so I hope my son's story helps someone out there. Here are some tips I wish I would have known:

ICE and cryo-are detrimental to nerves, bad for CRPS, heating blanket when cold.

MOVE- it hurts but, keep moving, being immobile makes you more immobile.

PT as early as you can, every little bit will help you get further, Water PT is even better!

Try not to rely on walkers, wheelchairs, do your best PT to stay mobile. Counseling- If you are in chronic pain and depressed get help, talk to someone.

Pain pills, gabapentin-in our case I wish we would not have used these at all or as long as he did. Honestly, if you can try treatments like Calmare and HBOT that are painless before medications. This is a personal choice, but it's one of the biggest regrets I have.

Consider diet changes and research supplements. Austin takes Fish oil, R-Lipoic Acid, and B complex (for nerve health), Turmeric (anti-inflammatory), Vitamin C (for no CRPS spread or recurrence) and Neuro Mag (magnesium- calcium channel blocker).

If a new surgery is needed for an unrelated condition, take vitamin C before and after surgery (50-days total-we use 1000 mg time-released). Also, read up on anesthetic protocols to help prevent CRPS spread. A ketamine infusion during surgery and an epidural nerve block could help as well. Consult with your doctor and the anesthesiologist before any procedure.

If you are a caregiver or loved one, be understanding of the pain your loved one is feeling. Be supportive and be present. Our son was a teen and when we should try to let him be more independent, we were babying him. We learned to stop asking constantly about his pain. Asking about pain reminds people they are in pain. As he got better, we tried to give him chores he could do and allow him to be more independent even though we wanted to coddle him.

Other therapies that Austin thought were helpful-mirror therapy, Epsom salt foot baths, rice tub for desensitization, red light therapy.

Occasionally, Austin feels shocks in other parts of his body, it's not spread. He gets up and moves around, and it goes away. Don't stress about it, just move!

As difficult as this CRPS situation was for our son and our family, we were fortunate to find some great doctors:

His surgeon Doctor Ty Endean, we are grateful for his quick diagnosis as a delay in proper diagnosis can be even more detrimental to treatment or possible remission.

Doctor Jonathan Tait from Rejuv Medical Southwest for his dedication to treating our son, his compassion and genuine care for Austin's best health. This doctor is one of kind and a blessing to anyone in his care. He believes in looking at alternative treatments for rare conditions and overall health.

Doctor Michael Cooney for his knowledge of CRPS and expertise in Calmare and helping patients worldwide.

Doctor Ryan Wade for his knowledge of CRPS and Calmare treatments.

The swelling and color changes were noticeable from the first month. The color improved with HBOT, but was still apparent when he had his leg down (not elevated). The rash appeared after he began using ketamine cream and lidocaine patches for the pain spot he had on top of the foot. This rash was a huge concern for months as we were afraid of infection. Epsom foot baths helped, however after Calmare the rash and lesions completely went away. He has had no recurrence of the rash or lesions since Calmare. He no longer uses the Rx cream or patches. He was able to wear socks and shoes after Calmare. Both legs and feet are now the same color and no swelling. Please view the following pictures.

"I WISH I HAD CANCER"
By: Joi Suissa

This story is about my son Justin Suissa who had reflex sympathetic dystrophy (RSD). He was 35-years-old when he committed suicide. He was extremely intelligent and talented. He attended Carnegie Mellon. He started a web design company. That's what he was doing when he took his life. Unfortunately, this autoimmune disease drove him to take his own life. He had the pain and frustration for about five years, which started at the beginning of 2011. It took him two years to be diagnosed. I'm not even sure if Justin really could pinpoint what happened. He came back from a trip to Switzerland and didn't feel great. He also thought he injured himself running.

Slowly the symptoms started to appear. Justin kept saying he couldn't have a blanket touch him.

He had trouble wearing shoes and jeans. He couldn't even have a feather touch him. At this time, we thought he should try to go to the Mayo Clinic. I thought it might be good to be examined there. When they told him, he didn't meet the criteria Justin started to look for an RSD specialist. Every day was torture for him. Justin had pain in different parts of his body. He had been to doctors that were supposed to be the top in their field. Basically, no one could pinpoint what was causing this pain. He had been in and out of every emergency room in every hospital in Manhattan. In the middle of the night, he took a cab to the emergency room again. This time, an intern there told him what he thought it was. The intern said it was an autoimmune disease called RSD. At work, I found a broker whose daughter had RSD. All the symptoms were exactly the same. His daughter was being treated at Boston Children's Hospital. Being a child, she was in control of her disease. Her treatment was successful. She eventually went on to college.

One of the biggest problems was that Justin's father didn't believe any of his symptoms. His father took him to a doctor that was supposed to be the best in Manhattan. Maybe, he was as an excellent doctor, but he didn't know anything about RSD. Then, slowly Justin's mouth started to hurt, so he went to the dentist. I couldn't tell you how many trips he made. It was exhausting to even catch a cab while he was in severe pain. He was given so many drugs I couldn't even tell you what they were. It is ridiculous to me that a person who can barely move about, had to go in person to get his meds. The meds were a control substance. The whole procedures made no sense. It was so frustrating to Justin. Now his teeth were being worked on. The pain in his body was horrible. He could barely put clothes on. His shoes hurt. Finally, he began searching on his own for a doctor. He found Doctor H., an RSD specialist on 72nd Street. He said he specialized in RSD. Justin went there on a regular basis to get a shot under his arm. He also was given some prescriptions. Doctor H., also explained a procedure in South America. They put you in a coma. The outcome could be brain damage or a permanent coma. There are two wonderful choices.

After reaching out to a lot of people Justin connected with the President of RSD memberships. One-month Justin got an invite to a meeting in the city with people all over the country who have RSD. There he met a woman who became a lifeline for Justin. Unfortunately, she lived in Michigan. She was married with children. I think they spoke daily for hours every day.

Justin also had one or two other people he shared his painful situation with. Justin always said, because he lived alone and was not married, he had no incentive to live. I begged him constantly to live with me. He did not want to be on Long Island.

He felt he would never see his friends. He also at this point had a team of doctors in Manhattan. After looking into many options, he decided to try a spinal cord stimulator (SCS). It was a Medtronic stimulator.

Another friend sufferer had pushed him to switch doctors and do the stimulator elsewhere. As Justin's luck would have it (something he complained about all the time) he had no luck. The day of his surgery, we had Super Storm Sandy. He had to stay with his partner family. She was a lovely woman with two children and a husband on 65th Street. Imagine being in that situation and being in pain. Every event in the Tri-State area affected Justin in some way.

Even, something as simple as a street closing or a parade. One of his fellow sufferers was very successful in getting him ketamine compound pain lotion. It would help him with numbing and desensitizing the pain caused by RSD. Even something as simple as getting his prescription was a nightmare. Of course, it was another drug not covered by insurance. His lotion was originally $300. At this point, it allowed him to tolerate wearing clothing and shoes. Basically, he always told her nothing helped. Justin was never a positive person. The cream did help him.

Suddenly, the cream went up to $600 a tube. He was smart enough to look up the properties of the cream. He was able to custom order it from a South Carolina company. This medicine was also not covered by insurance. He ordered the most effective properties for a lot less money. It seemed like any medicine relieve his pain wasn't covered. Then, there was the visit to his dermatologist. He had all different kinds of rashes and irritations constantly. Justin found a Doctor S., whom he respected and loved. This doctor was not covered by his insurance.

He had his own web design business. This always enabled him to work from home. That turned out to be a blessing because he could have never held down a job. He was sleeping a good part of the day and working at night. I don't know how he even did that. As time went by, his eyes were giving him a problem. The eye doctor gave Justin some special eyewear. It seemed as if something different was wrong every day. Justin looked into a special treatment performed only in Staten Island at a facility. I took him there for a few visits. I never really understood how this was going to help his pain. Of course, you know it didn't help. Like a lot of treatments, it seemed like a scam. I would take Justin to anything he wanted to try at this time he also started to use a cane. That did not sit well with him. He talked about suicide all the time. He said he wished he had cancer because then people would feel sorry for him. Justin looked well to someone on the outside. He was terrified to become wheelchair bounded. One of the women that had RSD had a lot of the same complaints as Justin.

Whenever he went anywhere to meet a friend or have someone over, he claimed that he paid the price for a few hours of fun. His last outing was to attend the wedding of one of his best friends. His friends brought him a tuxedo, shirt, shoes and all. He was in the wedding party. He tried his best to stay the entire wedding, but he couldn't. It would take weeks for him to feel better. He started to feel it wasn't worth to leave the house. One of the women who had RSD was religious. Her faith keeps a positive a very different positive outlook. She has faith. He didn't want to live this way. There were times I could see his point. I never wanted his life to turn out this way. His brother was upset when he got married across the country that Justin didn't attempt to be at the wedding.

I offered to take him and have someone help us, but he turned down the offer. His brother thought for sure he would try to kill himself that weekend. Sometimes, he basically was off the grid for the weekend. That's when I knew he was doing some powerful illegal drug to kill the pain. He didn't work or answer any calls when he did that. I spent years worrying when he didn't communicate with us, he killed himself. Justin had not spoken to his father for years.

When he did appear in Justin's life, he offered the most ridiculous things he thought Justin needed. One time, he offered Justin a grill for his terrace. Justin lost his mind. He was screaming at his father that his hands were shaking and could barely hold utensils. Did his father think he was going to take the tank to get gas? That was the help he offered. He was a wealthy man with no empathy.

January 2016

A few days into January, Justin said he didn't feel right. By night time, he got in a cab and went to the NYU emergency room. He was admitted right away. Justin had a triple pneumonia. He was in ICU for months. One day, they took him down to the operating room for some test. Always making sure he had a DNR. It was heartbreaking to hear that. Whatever they did, it was so painful, he said he's never doing that again. Of course, with Justin's luck, they had done it again. I knew he wished he would die from the operation or test. That would have been easy to explain to everyone. Finally, they took him out of ICU. I think this last hospital visit did him in. He swore he was never going to be in a hospital again. When he got out of ICU, his brother flew in from California to help him. After getting out from NYU, they wanted to send someone who would help him at home. Of course, he wouldn't accept the help. That was my son. I kept coming to help as much as I could. I worked and lived on Long Island. Soon, it was May and he appeared to be getting better. I picked him up for Mother's Day. He was going to spend the weekend. Justin was not only on time, which he hadn't been since he got sick. He was outside nicely dressed with flowers. He didn't complain about the drive out to the Island. The whole weekend was the best Mother's Day I had in years. I drove him home, not realizing it would be the last time I would see him. I could never have imagined losing a child no less to suicide. You know the saying "A mother should not bury a son." To this day I can't believe he is gone. He passed away on May 22, 2016. I wrote this story in the loving memory of my son Justin.

MY LIFE LIVING WITH VENIPUNCTURE CRPS II
By: Tracy Jones

My, name is Tracy Jones and in June of 2001, my life, as well as my husband, and my boy's (ages 7 and 10) would be changed from the way we had always known it to be. I went to the Emergency Room for kidney stones; however, I left the hospital with a disease called complex regional pain syndrome (CRPS), also known as reflex sympathetic dystrophy (RSD).

When I went to the hospital for the kidney stones, I received an I.V. in my right arm. I was told that they were going to give me some medicine through the I.V., so that I could pass the kidney stones. When the nurse started putting the medication into the I.V., it started burning. I asked if this was common and she said yes.

The next day, my right arm that the I.V. was put into was throbbing. Later that day I became very nauseated and my hand started swelling. My husband took me back to the hospital, and we were told that it was fine that when they put the I.V., in, it just infiltrated the vein and it will be fine. The swelling never went away and my hand stayed very red. I tried to hide how much pain I was in from my family; however, after several months, I finally made an appointment with my primary care doctor. My primary care doctor told me it could take up to six months for the redness and swelling to go away and that the pain I was describing could not be true. He did an X-ray which did not show anything wrong with my hand or arm even though you could feel knots on my arm where the vein when up to where the I.V., was placed.

Over the next five months, I saw two primary care doctors who told me that all I wanted was pain medication; however, one of the doctors decided to send me to a neurologist. I was so excited that he was going to refer me because I believed that maybe that doctor could help me. The neurologist did a nerve conduction test that only made by pain worse and then told me that maybe I have Carpal Tunnel from being a dental assistant. I advised him that I was only a dental assistant for about a year and the pain did not start until after I had received an I.V. for kidney stones.

I was still in so much pain and could not get any help from any doctors. Finally, in January of 2002, I went to see my gynecologist and I showed her my hand. She was very concerned and made me an appointment with a hand specialist that took another two months to get an appointment with.

I remember on the way to the appointment to the hand specialist just praying to Jesus that he would believe me and that I was not making all of this up. The doctor came in and asked me about my symptoms and how I had hurt my hand. As I was talking, he started looking at my hand and now my arm was starting to spread up to my elbow. He then said, "I know what you have, it is called Reflex Sympathetic Dystrophy (RSD)."

The doctor recommended that I have a stellate ganglion block (SGB) and said that this nerve block should help control my pain. He had given me a pamphlet on RSD to read, and he also recommended that I should do an online search on RSD, to educate myself about the disease. As I walked out, he said: "I'm sorry you have this condition and it is going to change your life forever." As I got into my car, I could no longer hold back my tears, I finally had a diagnosis and confirmed that RSD is a real condition. I had several SGB performed, which did help me for a while to manage my pain, for the next ten months.

During those ten months, I continued to work as a dental assistant; however, in March of 2003 I was at work when a piece of machinery came down on my thumb on my right hand and now the pain was worse than it was before I had received the two-nerve block. I made another

99

appointment with the hand specialists which took over three weeks to get in to see him and by then I was in so much pain that I could hardly stand it.

The doctor said that after having a second trauma to my hand was not good. He did another nerve block to see if it would help with the pain. The nerve block was not working this time, so he sent me to physical therapy, but that did not help either.

I finally had to quit my job because the pain was so unbearable that I could not sleep and I was throwing up all the time. I was finally sent to a pain management doctor who tried several other types of nerve blocks, but still could not get any relief. He suggested a tens unit. I did this and got some relief, but not enough to help with the pain. He later suggested that I try a trial stimulator that can later be inserted into your back. We did the trial simulator and I felt some relief. It is now August of 2003 and I went back to work and I'm trying to work with the trial simulator on my arm; however, the pain is so bad and I now have a tremor in my right hand that I finally had to quit my job. I had to wait until December of 2003 to get approval to get the actual stimulator inserted into my back. The stimulator helped; however, I continued to have so much pain in my hand and arm up to my shoulder and then down to my right leg.

In 2004, I was having more pain and swelling in my hand, arm, and leg. My leg was getting worse and it was swelling about an inch larger than my left leg. I was also starting to have tremors in my leg. The tremors in my leg are not all of the time; however, the hand tremors never stop. My hand is constantly shaking. If I get upset it shakes even more. My doctor is now not sure how to help me so he sends me to another pain management doctor who changes some of my medicines; however, still, no relief from the pain and he knew of no other options for me. So, in June of 2005, he decides to send me to another pain management doctor who has only been in Oklahoma for about two weeks. I started researching again about

RSD and found information concerning Ketamine Infusions for RSD patients that were being done in Germany.

The day, I met my new pain management doctor, he asked me if I knew about the Ketamine Infusions that were being done to help RSD patients? I knew at that very minute that Jesus had answered my prayers with a doctor who knew more about RSD than any of the other doctors that I had seen in the past and he was the closest answer to a cure or at least the closest person that could help me (truly a godsend to me). I went on an oral dose of Ketamine to see how that would help me. It did not do much, but we tried an outpatient trial of the Ketamine, which helped for about a day.

By the summer of 2005, everything changed for me. I've had RSD for five years and now, it is starting to affect my organs. I had my gallbladder removed, had another kidney stone that had to be removed by lithotripsy. The doctor informed my family that the procedure was done and everything went well, so he was leaving for the day. When I woke up, I was in so much pain and since the staff did not know anything about RSD just kept saying that it was the RSD causing the pain. I kept trying to explain to them that I know the difference between RSD pain and other pain. The pain that I was feeling was on my left side, not my right side. My family was beside themselves because I was thrashing and the doctors and nurses said that they could not do anything. They finally admitted me into the hospital and got my pain under some control. They did a CT scan and I was bleeding from my kidney so that led to a five-day stay in the hospital. All this suffering because most doctors and nurses don't listen to the patient.

After getting over the bleeding, kidney, I started gaining weight for no reason. I had not changed my eating habits (which because of the pain, I do not eat very much). Like always I started researching on the computer to try to see what was happening to me. What I found was Doctor Hooshmand's RSD Puzzles book and it asked if anyone received RSD from an I.V... I responded that I had received RSD through an I.V... I received a printout back about how getting RSD from this type of injury (known as Venipuncture CRPS II) is a one in a million chance and that this is the worst way to get it because it affects the blood vessels to the organs as well.

By now I am no longer sleeping in the same bed as my husband. I am either propped up on the couch or in the recliner. Unless there is a cure, I will never be able to sleep in a bed again.

The pain is now starting to be throughout my whole body. By 2007, my stomach is so swollen that I look like I'm pregnant, so I go back to my gynecologists who did an ultrasound and informs me she is pretty sure I have ovarian cancer. I have surgery and my ovaries are removed and thankfully there is no cancer. My ovaries were so inflamed that they looked like they had tumors on them. I thought that this was the problem; however, I continued to feel bad and in May 2007 they found a nodule on my thyroid. They did a biopsy and ran blood work and told me I was fine, not to worry even though I had every symptom that goes along with hypothyroidism, such as my hair falling out, losing my eyebrows, my feet hurt so bad I can stand to touch the ground and I can't stay awake. I was just told to stop eating. No one would listen to me.

Also, while all of this is going on, I am now watching my face cave in on my left side. What started as an indentation on the top of my cheek is now progressing to now look as if I have a sunken in check. I have now been diagnosed with another rare orphan disease called Parry-Romberg Syndrome.

After a lot of research between myself, and my pain management doctor, we diagnosed this and we found a correlation that shows Parry-Romberg Syndrome is affected by the sympathetic nerve so this ties back to the RSD. I went to the Mayo Clinic and they gave me a definite diagnosis of Parry-Romberg Syndrome. They only thing that they could help me with was the diagnosis and that I have a complicated medical history. I have also been diagnosed with Ankylosing Spondylitis which is another autoimmune disease which means my lower back is fusing together. I was also diagnosed with Fibromyalgia at the same time. I have done a lot of research that indicates that people are being told that they have Fibromyalgia really have Hypothyroidism. I can tell you that when my thyroid medicine is not working properly, I am in so much pain during that time. I had a friend tell me one time that when my medicine is not working, I look like I'm 80-years old, but when it is working, I look the age that I am.

In May of 2011, I had to have my appendix removed, but as usual, I had to have my I.V., put my foot since the veins are gone in left arm and my right arm cannot be used because of the RSD. The surgery could not be the simple type of surgery, they had to cut me open because my intestines had so much swelling and infection that could not see my appendix to remove it. I was in the hospital for five days. While in the hospital, signs were hung around the room stating that no one could touch my right arm, nor use it to take my blood pressure. The nurses would always try to use my right arm for getting my blood pressure and totally ignored the signs. The nurses knew nothing about RSD and in the beginning, after the surgery, I needed help to get out of the bed to go to the bathroom. When I tried to explain to the nurse that she could not pull or touch my right arm to help me, her response was "Well, I guess your family needs to help you" and walked out of the room instead of trying to learn how to help an RSD patient. Someone from my family had to stay with me 24- hours a day. After all of this, I had a horrible reaction to some blood pressure medicine that caused me to have hives all over my legs and torso. It is the summer and we are setting records for the number of days over 100 degrees, so I couldn't wear shorts since my legs looked so bad and it took two rounds of steroids to help; however, I now have scars on my legs.

It is now September of 2011 and I am starting to tell that my thyroid is not working properly again and my stomach is hurting just like before when I had my appendix removed. I go back to the doctor and they run blood work and a CT and I am told that everything is fine and she will see me in eight weeks. Since the doctor is only relying on the blood work and I am hurting, I finally demanded that she send me to a gastroenterologist. She referred me to a gastroenterologist who did a scope and found that I have ulcers exactly where I told him I was hurting.

By now, it has been five weeks for me to find out that I have ulcers and I know that my thyroid is not working properly. I have become very hoarse all the time. I go see my endocrinologist who does blood work and then feels my thyroid. He wants me to do an ultrasound the next week. I get my blood work back and he does the ultrasound and finds out that the nodule on the right side is still growing even though I have been on thyroid medicine.

The doctor wants to do a biopsy which will take another week and it shows no cancer and he doesn't know why the nodule is growing (I know why the thyroid is growing it is because of the RSD). So now I am going to a surgeon to see about getting the thyroid removed and also, I have to have a port put in because all of my veins are gone from only having one arm to use for any blood work or blood pressure. As well, it is known for CRPS to spread from any needle stick and it is now taking up to five to six sticks for blood work and sometimes they can't even get the blood. I have my thyroid removed and have a port put in.

After six years of trying all kinds of thyroid medicine and nothing was working, I started researching about the thyroid and asked the doctor to test for RT3 hypothyroidism. My doctor agreed to run the tests and it turns out that my hypothyroidism is called RT3 hypothyroidism which is rarely tested by doctors.

Also, in 2016 I had to have my spleen removed. Now, most of my organs have been removed from having CRPS.

In 2017, I was diagnosed with another rare disease called Gastroparesis, which is linked to someone having RSD.

I've been trying hard to raise awareness for CRPS as this is a horrible condition. I started a support group in 2009 to raise awareness and support for CRPS. From 2009 to the present the Oklahoma Governors have signed a Proclamation for November to be CRPS Awareness Month. The City of Mustang, Oklahoma in which I live, also does a Proclamation for CRPS Awareness Month. I would love to be able to get an Oklahoma bill passed for research and awareness for CRPS. Other states have already done this, but we could be one of the first states in the central part of the United States to do this. We need this so desperately! I've not been to an emergency room or to a hospital where one nurse knew what CRPS was unless a patient before me or a friend or family member had CRPS.

Because doctors and nurses aren't familiar with CRPS, I've been told that I must be a former drug addict since my veins are so bad and because of the pain medicine, I am on. People believe I am addicted. This is not the truth; I need this medicine the same way a diabetic needs insulin. I had someone tell me, "well at least you don't have cancer." If I had cancer, there would be a whole team of doctors working to make me better, but with chronic pain, this is not the way it is. This needs to be changed, the problems with all of the drug overdose from pain medicine are horrible, but the research shows that people with chronic pain are not addicted or abusing pain medicine.

We are the ones who are being a victim of this. Some CRPS patients are being denied their medicine because of the pill-pushing doctors and the drug abusers.

In Summary

My CRPS developed from a Venipuncture injury (I.V. needle) which is one in a million chance that this will occur. I didn't know for over nine months what was wrong, I only knew that the pain in my right hand was the worst pain I have ever had and the swelling was so bad that I couldn't close my hand at times, and the color changes from red to purple. I went to doctor after doctor trying to get help to only be told it must be phlebitis from the I.V., and it will go away.

That this disease would turn into a devastating disease that is the most painful thing you can have on the McGill Pain Index. The pain is worse than natural childbirth, worse than cancer unless the last stage in which you are given high doses of pain medicine.

I've had to mourn my life before CRPS and start a new life that is not easy. My children were very young when I received this disease and I would have to say to them "no I can't play ball with you; no, I can't push you on the swing and no I can't hold you or let you touch my right arm." I've also had to learn how to do things slower and with a different attitude.

I am very fortunate to have a loving husband, children, parents, sisters, aunts, etc., that are always there for me and to support me to help me with this horrible disease.

Please help me to share my story so that I can help others with this horrible disease. November is our Awareness Month for CRPS. I'm just trying to help anyone who is suffering from this disease. My support group is now on Facebook under: Oklahoma RSD/CRPS.

CRPS AND ME: THE PAINFUL TRUTH!
By: Michelle Engbrock

Complex regional pain syndrome (CRPS), the crappiest, lying, thieving disease out there. Never did I ever think I would be sitting here telling my story of a lifetime pain that was started from a small surgery. But here I am about to share the start, the lies that doctors tell you or want you to believe, friends and family who "THINK" they have had pain and you just got to take a Tylenol and it's gone. Or my favorite one, it's all in your head!! You're a simple psychological case looking for attention! Well, I wish it were just that easy, you know to turn it on and off at my own will for that attention that people think I'm seeking.

So how did I get here? In 1995, I had foot surgery. It was supposed to be a simple surgery and nothing more. By trade, I'm an Oral Surgery Assistant which as my profession, I'm on my feet all day every day. Doing that is very hard on the feet regardless of how good your shoes are. And a secondary factor, I was overweight too. So, two strikes against my feet. Over time I developed what they call Plantar fasciitis. It is a tendon/muscle group on the bottom of your foot. It's the area that burns when you have walked or run too much. Most people get past it, but a lot who are in a profession of standing get it and there are not too many options.

Every single day getting out of bed to start my day just hurt. It hurt to walk, stand or even stretch my feet. The only time my feet didn't hurt was when I was laying down. Over time of just trying to suffer through it, it got worse. Now my ankles were given out, it felt like I was standing on rocks all day. My legs were swollen and at the age of 26, I was miserable! I was supposed to be able to go to work, go home and do fun stuff with my husband, not want to just lay down. So, after trying to handle this on my own without much success I decided I needed to go see a foot specialist. If anyone knows about us people in the medical field, we hate and I mean hate going to doctors. We know too dang much and we tend to get a little bossy. But I needed this pain gone because trying to stand in the operating room or just walking to my car was becoming too painful. Crawling everywhere was looking quite appealing.

I went to see a foot doctor or podiatrist for some help. The one I had originally wanted to see was unavailable, but his partner had openings. The staff assured me he was a wonderful person and would get me functioning again. Well, I was ready! I met this doctor and my first impression was... he was ok. He was older, grandpa type, but says he has 30 plus years of experience. So, I get X-rays, and my feet poked on and measured, etc... That's when he told me I had plantar fasciitis and, in most cases, a few steroid shots and a little physical therapy would fix me right up. But if not, the next option is to get custom shoe inserts to help cushion and position my foot correctly since I had been walking on the sides of my feet because of the pain. And if all that didn't work, then surgery, which would cut that fascia or tendon type thing in the middle of my foot so it could no longer spasm or tighten up causing pain. So, we started all the conservative treatments, and nothing was helping. The doctor at the time seemed to truly care about helping the pain. But after trying the steroid shots in my feet, which by the way were painful in itself, if you think getting a shot in your arm is painful, think again.

Someone sticking this 2-inch needle in the side of your foot and ankle...ha! I'm a strong person, I work with blood and all the other yucky stuff in my profession, I don't faint at the sight of disgusting things.

But that shot, whew, that brought me to a level of never again! Even though the shots worked at first, they didn't last long. So, it was the decision to go forward with surgery because of my profession of being on my feet that seemed to be the best option since all else failed long term.

Now being in the medical field I tend to think I'm cautious. I asked questions, I researched his record through the medical board, looking for malpractice claims. Nothing! Things seemed all was okay with this doctor that I was about to trust my feet too. The surgery was supposed to be simple day surgery. A little sedation and I go home and recover. According to him, I should be back in my shoes in seven to ten days and for the most part pain-free within a month. Just soreness that physical therapy would take care of. My surgery day was approaching and my nerves were on edge, but no turning back, I wanted to walk without this pain. I had the surgery on both feet so it would be done and over with. A piece of advice.... Never do both feet at the same time. So, I'm in recovery with both feet bandaged and in those funky surgery shoes and crutches. Oh, yeah! These boot things with ice to keep the swelling down and the best part, good pain meds. Time to recover! I took two weeks off from work to recover and try to be the model patient. I went to my first post-op visit five days after surgery.

The doctor is asking how it was going? Well, I was still having this throbbing pain and still needing the stronger pain meds. He tells me I need to start physical therapy and try to get off the strong pain meds. I start physical therapy and try to get through this pain. But according to the doctor, I shouldn't be having pain like this and I needed to get tougher. Okay, so maybe I was a bit soft or so I thought, but dang this was incredibly painful, nothing like what he told me it would be. I continue my PT and still hurting. So, he says it's time to start putting my tennis shoes back on and just walking and stretching. I did try, but this pain just wouldn't get easier. My two weeks off from work was up and I had to return to work. I wasn't sure how I was going to make it through the day but I would try. I was still taking mildly strong pain medication to help through the day. But by the end of the day, I was in agony. My legs were swollen, so much I thought I was going to have to cut my scrubs off me. I came home and elevated my feet and iced them, I did everything I knew to do, but nothing was helping.

I returned to the doctor and his attitude started to change towards me. Kind of blaming and condescending. I wasn't sure why, but just maybe I was being a big baby; I don't handle pain well, but this was just too much. The doctor said more therapy and I shouldn't have pain if I was doing as I was told, which I was. I did another month of physical therapy and sand therapy to help with the hypersensitivity to touch my skin. But this freaking pain wasn't getting better, it was getting worse. It was burning, I felt like my feet were on fire. I couldn't stand even socks to touch them. Walking, oh geez, I only thought the start of my original foot pain, hurt, nope, this was 10-times more painful. The odd thing was the outside of my feet the skin felt cold. I felt like I was standing on a nest of Hornets. By now I'm six weeks post-surgery and I'm having more pain than I can imagine, and I still can't put my shoes on as the doctor instructed.

I decided it was time to go see the doctor again. I told him about the pain and he is shaking his head, he asks why I have bandages on still. I told him that even though my feet feel like they are on fire, the outside is cold and I can't stand stuff touching them and this was my best option. The doctor who I thought seemed very concerned about me, has now turned into Doctor Jekyll and Mr. Hyde. He starts yelling at me to quit faking this pain for attention and drugs. He takes the surgery shoes I was wearing and throws them across the room. All I could do was ask him why am I still hurting? He said to me, you're not, it was now all in my head! I gather up my stuff and left feeling pretty helpless. What was I going to do now? I continued trying to work, but I was just exhausted from all the pain and trying to hold it together. My co-worker was having some foot issues too, and she suggested I go see her doctor for a second opinion. I agreed because I needed help. This was almost five months post-surgery and nothing was getting better.

I went to see the new doctor, but was very cautious again. I refuse to let some male doctor tell me I was crazy and making up this pain. So, I tell this doctor all that I was experiencing, pain, etc....and the poor doctor experience I had prior. He first says to me that what I'm experiencing he has seen come from this doctor over and over. In other words, mistakes! So, he tells me that because of what he knows about this doctor the best course of action is to do exploratory surgery and figure out what was going on. Well, I had no choice; surgery was scheduled and here we go again.

I remember this part so vividly. I'm undergoing this exploratory surgery and the doctor wakes me up from anesthesia to talk to me. He said to me that my feet are severely messed up and that fixing them in one surgery wasn't going to happen, so he was starting with one at a time and did I want him to continue? I remember saying yes, just get me out of pain and back off to sleep I went. I woke up in the recovery room and here is when I hear the dreaded news. It appears that whatever surgical instruments they used not only cut the plantar fascia but other structures as well like my Achilles tendon and left a ton of scar tissue that had nerves going thru it and this was going to take a series of surgery and be placed in a pair of special surgery boots etc, in hopes to fix it. All I could do was cry and agree to hopefully get me fixed. He said he hopes that with this surgery, he could put me back together again. I went through six surgeries to fix this incredible mess. But this burning pain never left. The spasming and twitching of my toes stopped, but not the burning pain. But this doctor who put me back together starts telling me that he thinks now that I'm internally fixed because it was a mess, he says with the symptom of burning I might have another issue, but this one may not be fixable. That's when he asked me if I had heard of reflex sympathetic dystrophy (RSD) before? I told him that I heard of it before. I had a patient with it in their arms and they told me about the burning and unending pain. He mentioned to me that he suspected that this is what I have. I was finally diagnosed with RSD in 1997. I asked him if it was from the original surgery? He told me yes, that surgery, trauma can cause it and the type of trauma or should I say the mess my feet were left in could have activated it. I asked him if all these other surgeries would have added to it, he says no but it certainly did not help. He said I did not have an option to not fix it. I was literally in a wheelchair and without fixing, it I wouldn't walk again. He gave me the info and told me that basically, we are entering a new journey together and that he was not going to leave me, but he would help me find the right doctors to help me. He told me it was time for me to go educate myself on this so I could make informed decisions. I was stunned, now what? I was newly married, and we were trying to adopt a baby. I had to put all my dreams on hold for now. If anyone is wondering if I was still working? The answer is yes, but barely!

I was wearing surgery boots 24/7 and in horrible pain and trying to make it through each hour. Lunch couldn't come fast enough so I could try to nap through my day. I had to learn to sit during surgery and re-adapt my techniques of practice. I was also missing a lot of work to get X-rays, cat scans, bone scans, and the list goes on. My foot doctor first sent me to a pain management doctor because my pain needed to be handled on a higher level than what he had experience for. He found all the doctors involved in my care to make sure I was getting the best care and yet standing by my side.

My next stop was to see the pain management doctor. Now, I've never been one to take lots of medications, but I was ready to take anything to help stop this pain. He first put me on morphine. Well, that helped, but the side effects were horrible. I had itching, nausea, and severe headaches. So, on to the next drug, Dilaudid, and some other pain medications that were alternated. Now, I was in a drug zone, even though the pain was still there, and the euphoria from the drugs had me on a different plane. Since I was in the medical field, I was fully aware of what these drugs could do to my liver. I stayed atop of the blood testing for my liver and kidneys. But as the days and years passed me wanting to be a mom was still on my mind. How much longer would this be? At, the time I was diagnosed there weren't many treatments for RSD. The studies were just starting to come out. So, for me, all I could do was continue the pain medications. With all of this going on I did eventually lose my job and started sinking into a deep depression. I couldn't do anything but stay in bed and watch TV. Any friends I had started leaving because I was in pain and they didn't understand this level of pain.

You know everyone has experienced your kind of pain, and they just take medication and made it through. No, sorry this type of pain you have no idea what I'm going through. My family didn't understand why we wouldn't travel to see them. Simply, the vibration of the car sent my pain into overdrive! I had nothing left, but my two dogs who nursed me all day long. My mom tried to keep my spirits up, but she also hated seeing me so miserable. Crying became a daily thing. I felt like I had nothing to live for. So, did I question suicide? Maybe for a brief moment, I just didn't want more pain to do it and my dogs and husband and mom meant everything to me. So, I continued my fight!

I had a lot of appointments with the pain doctor, a lot of judgment looks from pharmacies as well as other doctors who had no clue what RSD was. I got accused of being a drug addict as well! The excitement just never ended! I finally asked my pain doctor was there any hope of me getting off these drugs! I hated them, but needed them. I wanted to be a mom, but how when I was under the influence of some big-time drugs. That's when he told me about a new study using a device called an intrathecal pain pump for chronic pain. He said he could sign me up if I was willing but that he would have to transfer my care to someone else. What did I have to lose? If it worked, I had a lot to gain! So basically, I was going to be the youngest person to go through a trial using the intrathecal pain pump, something that was traditionally used for end of life cancer patients. So, off to another doctor!

The next thing was getting set up for a trial for the intrathecal pain pump. If it worked, they would put one in after a few weeks, if it didn't then I don't know? My new doctor wanted to try two different things, the intrathecal pain pump and the spinal cord stimulator (SCS). He said if the trail of the SCS worked for me, it might be a better option to help control my pain because it works off electrical currents and not drugs. But if the pain pump worked, I had to understand that this is a lifetime commitment, you are "basically" married to your doctor. But I was ready because if this worked, I could try to get a little more control over my life and start the journey of becoming a mom.

Surgery day... I won't lie, I was terrified because surgery started all this pain. Another trauma or even surgery can cause RSD to spread to other areas. I woke up with both devices in place. The SCS was on and the pump was not, the catheter was in place. The SCS was a definite no go. After about six hours, I was in more pain and felt like it was a crawling pain up my legs. I turned it off and the next morning my doctor turned the pump on, and we decided to do a weeklong trial. It was amazing, my pain went from 10+ to about a five. It was the first time, in three years, I felt some hope. So, after my trial I had the permanent pump placed. I started coming off the hard-oral drugs because I didn't need them, that's what the pump is for. My doctors told me that even though I have this pump it is only a pain focused device and not everyone will understand how it works. But, with this pump I would also get some freedom back, I wouldn't be all doped up to the point of barely knowing my name.

The pump itself isn't perfect, but it has its issues too. Make sure you have a doctor who knows how to put them in and manage it. I had serious issues a few times with my first few pumps only because the doctor who did my trial was not going to be the doctor who would eventually put it in and manage it. I think I went through three doctors and problems after problems that I didn't think I would encounter. Spinal fluid leaks, drug withdrawal because they would forget to fill the pump and turn it on, seroma, the pump coming through my skin. I was ready to give up. My foot doctor stepped back in because remember he said he would be with me through my journey. He went to the doctor who did my trial and did the study as well as working with Medtronic's to help them with using this device for chronic pain. He told the doctor about my troubles and asked him to take me on as his private patient. He agreed to do so and he has been my doctor for the past 19-years.

I have had my pump since 1999. I will tell you that having this pump does have its complications. Doctors think they know how it works. They think it covers full-body pain, it doesn't. If I get a kidney infection, this pump will not help that pain. But try telling that to an ER doctor. All they see are drug seekers. So, going to see any doctor in the ER is a useless event, and trying to talk to a doctor who has a "God" complex is impossible. I try to avoid the ER if at all possible. I've had doctors tell me it affects my brain and response times with driving, no, it doesn't. I've had doctors tell me they cannot give me surgical pain meds because my pump drugs should be helping. I get so tired of doctors arguing that I've had back surgery, no my back is still intact. Yes, there is a scar, but that's where my catheter has been placed. My latest run-in with a big-headed doctor happened when they wanted me to have a myelogram done, which is a dye test in your spine while having an MRI. My response was I cannot have an MRI because it will damage my pump nor can you stick stuff in my spine because I have a catheter in my spine. The doctor said to me.... Oh, that's ok, we will work around it, I've seen them before. The key word is, "he has seen them before." Um no! This is something you don't pretend to know about because you have an MD behind your name. You can kill me with one bad move to my catheter. So, having this pump you have to be aware of everything and not trust doctors, they don't know, but that pride takes over regardless of putting the patient in danger. That's why I hate doctors who put these pumps in patients and then abandon them. That patient has a problem and they tell them to go to the ER. If a doctor wants to truly help us then they need to be there through the good and bad times. They need to stop looking at us as dollar signs!

But now I bet you are wondering about the doctor that started this mess? I did get an attorney and sued him. I found out later that he had done this before in another state. This other state doesn't make it public and that doctor left that state and came to my state and retook his license exam and was re-certified. But since he was a pro at this, he had put all of his assets in his kid's name so it couldn't be touched.

After getting hospital records, I found out that he allowed a student to operate unsupervised as well as not getting my consent. And the biggest one, he allowed his malpractice insurance to lapse one week before my surgery. The hospital unknown to me was in bankruptcy before my surgery, which eventually closed its doors because they had plenty of issues too. So, did I get anything from this lawsuit? No. The only satisfaction I got was taking his license away again and knowing he is now dead and can't hurt anyone again. As for me, well, I am permanently disabled, I'll always live in pain. My pain pump has been my saving grace. I did become a mom, but it hasn't been easy having chronic pain, but it gives me hope. I will always have pain and limited to what I can do. I can't work full time again; I can't enjoy amusement parks because my feet are destroyed, but functional enough to keep me out of a wheelchair.

My one hope is that doctors will learn about RSD/CRPS and take it seriously. Stop treating us like drug addicts. Stop taking our needed medications away because the government thinks they know best. I promise if someone working for the government went through the type of pain that we deal with every day they would be begging for something more than Tylenol. I hope one day they find a cure for CRPS, but until that time continue to advocate for yourself, teach the doctors and fight for our rights. I didn't ask for a botched surgery and life as I knew to be taken away from me. We are people too, and doctors must honor the Hippocratic Oath that they take to keep the patient from harm.

RSD BARBIE
By: Cindee Rose

My foot feels like I had smashed it in a door.

The pressure in my head, ugh... A woman outside my car window was saying, "whew, glad you're OK!"

Not concerned with myself, I had to look at my two-year-old son to ensure that he was "OK."

He is looking at me with his little eyes full of fear, saying "Uh oh you spilled our coffee!"

Mental note... Kiddo is OK... I think .... At least, he is not saying anything about any pain.

Now back to this woman... She frequently said, "My husband is going to kill me!" Now, she's worried about losing her clients.

However, it felt like my right foot and leg had been shoved into a meat grinder, and now my head was starting to throb.

OK! Next up, move this car... Protect my kiddo.

I move the car off the road, but my foot is now in excruciating pain. Thankfully, I was near my home...

The next few weeks were full of doctor visits. My foot was now flaming red and felt like I'd rather no longer have it attached to my body.

The podiatrist I was referred to put me in an air cast encasing my right foot so that I wouldn't put pressure on it. That lasted for six consecutive months. My busy life as a mom, VP of operations of a successful scrap metal business was slowly beginning to change.

The life I was living before this car accident happened, was slipping into memory. The amount of money I was spending was unreal. I had doctor bills after doctor bills. I began taking more and more personal time to research what was causing my pain.

I was so hell-bent on solving this, this current podiatrist kept telling me I must be getting better. Oh, must I?

No, sir, I was worse. Eight months later, he set me up in a new fancy Ballerina cast, gave me ibuprofen and continued to treat me with a new "ballerina slipper" every other week for another four months. After that failure, he then decided the next approach was to get a custom orthotic insert made for my shoe. I was then as I am now, I'll try most anything to try to help the pain. I was more thankful to be out of the casts. To no avail, it didn't help I continued to try to exercise through the pain trying to build my now weaker foot and leg back up. Many months spent sobbing while trying to create my "new normal."

By this time, it was two full years after my accident. My marriage was over, I wasn't working as I once was. I figured after seeing a multitude of doctors, four podiatrists, two orthopedic surgeons, and three family practice doctors, they were just thrown in for good measure I suppose. I decided to move to the Bay Area. A fresh start I figured would help my children, now ages 4 and 8 deserved it as well. My thought process was that of "its California" they must have more doctors there than in small little Washington. So off we went.

After going to my new family practice doctor, I was sent to a new Orthopedic surgeon. Another dead end.

Now, I had to begin seeing Physicians for the car accident case. I had to have an Electromyogram (EMG). This is a test that is used to record the electrical activity of the muscles. How to put it in layman's terms, it's a Frankenstein test. This doctor placed the needle electrodes into my muscles down through to the nerves in both arms and legs. Then, they flipped the switch to electrify my nerves. One by one my extremities shook uncontrollably. He continued this test for what seemed like 10-hours I was then told later it only took two and a half hours. That's the day I had my first seizure. I was so violently sick for the next three months. I was hospitalized and of course, the Physicians were clueless to what was wrong. I was sent home unable to walk. My legs would buckle underneath me when I tried to walk. I wish I could say that this was the only EMG that I needed to have, but unfortunately, it was followed by another with very similar results.

I had seen by this time another two handfuls of doctors. To say I was losing hope was an understatement, I was prescribed "medication cocktails" from Vicodin to aspirin to any narcotic and every under the sun. I refused to take them; it didn't make sense to add a band-aid to this problem at this point. I once had an extremely bad day reaction to one of these "medication cocktails", I'm included Effexor, I lost my memory. During this time, I even lost my memory. Not from narcotics from lack of sleep, food, and Effexor. The only reason I know what happened was from video footage my children (now 11 and 8) had taken. I was a shell of a woman 5'8 under 100 lbs.

My kids became my advocates, especially my daughter. As a Mom, my kids were still my greatest accomplishment. See I came from an extremely abusive set of parents. If it wasn't for my bonus Mom, I would never have seen nor known love. She still is the Mother I know God sent to me.

My kids learned my "ailment" thoroughly. They took care of so many daily things for me. They learned what it looked like if I was going to have a "seizure." My seizures don't look like epileptic episodes, they are tremors and do impair my speech.

Finally, in 2000, I was sent to a doctor that happened to attend the same college I did. Doctor T., was told about me and accepted the appointment to see me. She was a pain management doctor, which happened to have been newly diagnosed with Lyme disease. She took her time and evaluated me. She said, "I am not 100% sure what you have BUT I have a good idea. I'd like to begin working with you so I'm going to make some calls and see what I can do so that your insurance will allow that."

A long 48-hours later, she called and explained, I would need her as my primary physician for this to happen. She was a chronic pain management doctor, but she was what felt like my last hope. Over the next few months, she evaluated me. Then, the day came, I went to her office. After the usual pleasantries, she said it. I didn't hear it at first. Let's be real, after OVER FOUR long years of not knowing she could've said anything. The reality was I had AN ANSWER!

She said it again, "Cindee!" You have reflex sympathetic dystrophy (RSD)" She spelled it out for me." She said, the good news is this is what I believe you have.... The bad news there isn't a cure, but she said I will try like hell to help you maneuver and navigate it.

I broke into a million pieces. After four years of this and the lack of sleep, the constant pain, the stress itself of this terrible Bitch now dubbed RSD BARBIE... I had an answer.

My, kids and I always thought I should have an RSD BARBIE, so I could explain to people with a visual tool of sorts... Yes, I look like I look on the outside, but this horrible THING isn't pretty. I have often been told, "you don't look sick" or "you're too young and too pretty to be hurting as you claim."

Like I wanted to live this way. I do not sleep, and not to care for my kids at my absolute 100% best... Absolute Ignorance!!!

My doctor put me on Neurontin, and I believe along with my faith and my will, I know it has kept me going. I've had hyperbaric treatments that have helped also, thankfully those have dropped in price considerably since the first one way back almost 20-years ago.

I've learned many useful tools to help me cope with RSD. From yoga to refocusing my thoughts... To all things ice, yep ice is one of the worst things to use for us RSD vets. It's bad, and I do not recommend using it.

The pain in my lower back gets so excruciating that I have iced it and it has developed into third-degree burns. Once my back finally gets numb, it feels like it's been burnt. It's not numb, it's truly only a pissed-off RSD BITCH... There are actual blisters burnt on my skin... But for a few brief moments, my mind somehow thought it might not hurt as much as it does. Then I go through weeks of healing the burn. I don't sleep, which is extremely dangerous, I hurt 24/7 never is there a second without pain.

In those quiet moments at night, I try to focus on music or tv. Something to help me not think of how my body feels. I can't read for too long because my focus gets redirected to my pain too quickly. I can't read more than a paragraph... It's discouraging.

To be in a relationship with me is to be in a relationship with my RSD as well. She's (my RSD) is unkind and cruel to say I've had men leave me "us" because of it is an understatement.

It takes a strong man to stick by and live this life with me. I understand and accept it. My parents don't understand it. I don't blame them, my Dad, when he was alive, wanted me to "eat right for my blood type" believing if I did, I would be CURED...

I've been in remission twice, once in 2001 when my awesome doctor began treatment. Unfortunately, this remission was short-lived for only a few months. While I was exercising, I had collapsed, and my symptoms slowly began to return. The next time I went into remission was in 2008-2009 when I was pregnant with my youngest kiddo. Soon, after I delivered my son, the symptoms returned. Ten-years later remission lost its way to me.

To be raising another while having RSD present, I struggle. I have been denied disability numerous times. It's discouraging... So now fighting back with the knowledge to possibly help ANYONE I must say feels incredible! I must mention Eric Phillips, who through the years has been someone I have looked up to, for being a front-man in this band of members that would much rather be making music than being teachers of this cruel disorder. Thank you for lending us your voice, so we can be heard. No one truly understands what we have as he does. Bless people's hearts for trying to though.

HOPELESS NO MORE
By: Patty S.

I was driving home from work in April of 1993 and was the middle car of a three-car collision where my car was pushed into the car ahead of me. I was diagnosed with a concussion, whiplash, and a back sprain. I was treated with massages, physical therapy, muscle relaxers, and Naprosyn. Three months later, I developed severe right arm pain from my elbow to hand. My right hand to the elbow was swollen, sometimes my fingers would swell to three inches each and stiff. I had been seeing my primary care doctor, orthopedic, and neurologist. I had to wear a pad on my elbow to protect the nerves for six months, yet, the pad had increased the pain.

I had CT, MRI of my neck and elbow. I also had an EMG. I was sent to a psychiatrist and psychologist, because it was thought that the "pain was in my head." I started showing up at my primary care when my arm was purple and cold (without an office visit scheduled). I asked the doctors how was I making this happen? Was this in my head, too. I showed up at the doctor when my arm was burning, red and hot and told him I must have one powerful brain. I believe because, I was a successful pharmacist, doctors were listening to me. I gave them a list that detailed the pain (shocks from my elbow every 60 seconds that are worse than hitting one's funny bones. My arm was burning. It was not burning like a sunburn but burning like I put my arm on a burning stove) Had I been just a patient, I know they would have looked the other way. In the 1990s simply a little more was known about RSD than when it was first known during the civil war. Getting the information, the physicians need, takes an incredible amount of time (much more than the eight minutes allowed).

I was sent to a special neurologist (along with a normal neurologist), neurosurgeon, vascular surgeon, a special orthopedic surgeon, a psychiatrist, and a psychologist. I had a myelogram, SSEP, another EMG, also had some neurovascular test. I was told that my nerves were fine, my psychological profile was good, I simply had a low tolerance for pain, and I was not handling stress well, I needed to relax and take a vacation. They were willing to remove a rib even though I didn't have thoracic outlet syndrome (TOS) to improve the blood flow to my arm.

My primary care doctor believed me that I was in pain and sent me to a new neurosurgeon who read all these reports and is almost two years after the injury and 15 doctors later. He mentioned that this might be RSD? He sent me to another neurologist who agreed I had a "rare type of RSD." They recommended "the burn method." Doing this method, I had to use my hand and arm until it hurt so much I almost passed. I had to do this method four times a day for a month until "I burned the RSD out of me." This idea did not work at all and I became depressed.

During this time, I thought of suicide a lot and had come up with multiple plans. Seventeen doctors told me I would never be a pharmacist again, never work and I would be in constant pain for the rest of my life. I would never be able to use my right hand and ten years I would be confined to a wheelchair. No, part of me that wanted to live. NOT ONE DOCTOR offered me any type of hope. I tried overdosing on alcohol drank a 1/5 in an hour and threw up. I almost had enough pills saved up to end my life and I believe God intervened.

I told the psychologist they think I have RSD and there is no hope. He told me he went to a workers' compensation meeting where a physician who specializes in RSD talked and he gave me his name.

I called Doctor A.K.'s office to set up an appointment, and I needed a referral from two doctors. Primary care was easy, I showed up at the neurologist/neurosurgeon's office at 9:00 a.m. with donuts. I was told the first available appointment was in three months. For eight days, I brought donuts to the staff and stayed in the office from 9 a.m. to 4 p.m... Finally, the physician asked me what I was doing, I told him I found a doctor that

126

treats RSD and I need a referral from you and your next appointment is in three months so I am waiting for a cancellation. I had my referral the next day.

When I first saw Doctor A.K., he gave me a stack of papers telling me about RSD. He gave me some hope when he provided me with a game-plan. After six stellate ganglion blocks (SGB), I could move my hand and arm a little more and the pain was a little better (I went from an 8.5 to a 7). Part of the game-plan with Doctor A.K., was I had to prepare to go back to work. I was given a Thera-cane for muscle spasms and a tens unit. I had to desensitize my right hand, so I could hold a pen. I started pulling 10 weeds a day, three times a day and forcing myself to hold a pen. I also learned meditation. Holding a pen sounds so easy yet in the beginning, my hand would shake. Three months later, I had another round of six SGB. Six months later, I set up and started a free clinic pharmacy and less than a year later, I was working part-time. I was getting three SGB every four months, I wore a tens unit 15-hours a day and started taking Darvocet at bedtime.

In November of 1995, I jammed my right hand, and the RSD had spread to my shoulder. I had an SGB to help the pain, but it didn't work. In December of 1995, I had a right upper sympathectomy. After a tough recovery, I went back to work part-time. This might sound crazy, but I forgot about my right limb, it didn't hurt. (What I mean is when one is in constant pain you always know that limb is there, it hurts so much you can't forget it).

I was really down meeting with Doctor A.K., telling him I wished I could play volleyball, or go canoeing and do what 31-years old's do. He handed me this medical book and told me to look it up. Nowhere in this book did it say a pain management, patient couldn't play sports. He just told me not to dive for the ball and moderation was the key.

In 1997, I was in a car accident that ended up setting off the RSD on the top of my left hip to my foot and my right arm to my shoulder. (I had a CT of my head, neck, back, hip. I also had an MRI of my head, neck, back hip). I also had an EMG of my right arm and left leg. I was offered a left lower lumbar sympathectomy and opted for another round of three sets of three lumbar sympathetic blocks (LSB) and two sets of three SGB and was back in partial remission.

With mediation, relaxation techniques, and tens unit, I was able to return to work. I was on prn pain medication at bedtime, muscle relaxers. Yet working, living with pain does take an emotional/spiritual toll on your body.

There were many events that I would look forward to going to, but I had to cancel because of a bad flare that would prevent me from going. Over time, my friends stopped asking me out because I would say no, or I would leave too early. This can happen when CRPS takes over the brain. The loneliness, isolation, brokenness, and hopelessness can set in and I wanted to give up.

I was feeling anger, fear, depression and sometimes I felt I was the only one in the world with this disorder, which leads to days/nights of suicidal thoughts.

In 2004, I fell and broke my shoulder and damaged, both rotator cuff muscle. These two surgeries set off the RSD in my right arm, left leg and now left head to shoulder. Thank God my surgeon knew about CRPS, yet the pain was so intense for so long. Yet with the SGB and LSB, there was a "miracle drug" now used for sedation, it was Ketamine. I was given two sets of six left SGB, two Sets of three R-SGB and LSB. Each set was two months apart.

Ketamine with the blocks for me makes them last longer, and I love the feeling of not caring about the pain. In 2010, I was forced to retire because of CPRS in 75 % of my body. I became hypersensitive to sounds and smell.

My right arm and left leg stayed six degrees cooler than the rest of my body. With the help of a psychologist, I learned biofeedback.

Currently, I get two Ketamine Infusions every other year for full-body CRPS pain and when the pain is localized, I get SGB and LSB. I believe I have had over 150 R-SGB, 66 L-LSB, and 50 L-SGB. The problem I have now is that I need a shoulder replacement. Two physicians have told me to live with the pain because with the shoulder replacement and the narcotic situation, they will not be able to control the pain, and they don't want another patient killing themselves.

The annoying problems of dealing with CPRS to me is: being cold and sweating in Florida when its 88 degrees outside and I am in a light jacket. I don't like having to wear jeans outside when it's 90 degrees out, because the sun, and wind set off the pain in my leg. On a bad day when I get the tremor/shakes, people ask me if I have had too much to drink or I am simply trying to get attention, and people also tell me "that the pain can't be that bad, I should just get a job and the pain will go away" or "my" favorite line is that "God is punishing me for all my sins" (I answer how come murders don't have CRPS?). When it gets cold outside, anything under 70 degrees will set off my pain, and I can never get warm (my solution is, I always keep jackets in my car). With the hypersensitivity issues from the CRPS, I have had a hard time finding blankets and clothes I can wear. I finally found a furry dog blanket that I use because sheets hurt too much.

Living with CPRS is NOT for wimps, you will have unrelenting pain that starts in the day, and you toss and turn all night from the pain. Some bad days may last for a week or a month, and while other bad days will last only a day. Break down the bad days into 10 min sessions (after all anyone can deal with something for 10 minutes). I had to find people you can trust to talk about the pain and all the psychosocial issues. What has helped me is I have found places where I can volunteer.

What I learned when I am feeling suicidal, feeling overwhelmed, lonely, tired, a burden (to my family), broken and isolated is I should call a friend, or a support helpline, take a shower, take the dogs to the park, watch a movie, or watch a sunset, etc. (make up your plan before this feeling happens). Remember being suicidal is a feeling, just like being angry or sad. NO feeling, demands action and just like all feelings, they will pass.

My best tool for succeeding with CRPS is my attitude. Every morning, I try to find humor in each day, smile at strangers, watch my dogs play, and laugh. On bad days, I allow myself one hour to have a pity party.

When I started my RSD journey NO, ONE GAVE ME HOPE. When I went to the medical library to find information on RSD, I found out that it has been around since the civil war. Until I found Doctor A.K., I thought I was the only one with the rare disorder.

There is hope now, look at all the Facebook RSD/CRPS support groups: (RSDSA, International RSD Foundation, RSDHOPE, etc.) = you are not alone. New drug trials are going on today, just in Florida there are four. Many researchers are trying to find solutions. There are many dedicated and caring CRPS medical professionals trying to reduce suffering and make life better. There is a large clearing houses of CRPS information for you to learn about your disease.

SURVIVING RSD-CRPS WITH FAITH, HOPE, AND PRAYERS
By: Suzy Holcomb

On a crisp late Wednesday afternoon, around 5:45 p.m., the night before Thanksgiving in 1961, we were getting ready to enter our last Seventh Grade Science class of the day in middle school. We were on a split-session in our hometown, sharing the school with the high school students because some fellow in town attempted to set fire to the chemistry lab, nearly destroying the entire high school building. We only had a few more days to wait until the following Monday morning when we would be the first class to move into the brand-new middle school. Boy, were we excited! Hotshots we would be! As we approached our next class, in a circular fashion around the hall monitors, we were only a few short feet away from the doorway of our room, when this one boy who sat behind me in alphabetical order and who constantly irritated me, decided he would irritate me one more time. He decided on this night that he would stab me in my right forearm with a wooden pencil. I said what the heck just happened? Pain soared and blood spouted, as we stood right outside the Principal's office. To say the least, I never made it to class as my friends, teachers, and principal rushed me to the nurse's office. The pencil and lead had broken off inside my arm. The nurse did her best to clean the wound, removing what she could and called my Mom and Dad. We all headed directly to the doctor's office where he, in turn, entered the arm with a scalpel extricating the rest or most all the pencil and lead as possible. We were able to stop the bleeding. The pain was to beat the band. The swelling, redness, spasms, the feeling of pins and needles, daggers, and burning were the worst pain I have ever felt. I was given "light" pain medication due to my age and told to put ice on my arm due to the swelling. That hurt like Hell---o-----!

We were to attend a High School football game the next day and, of course, it was very cold outside. My pain levels were through the roof. I found out as the days went by that holding anything with this hand for any length of time, would become so distorted, deformed, and became quite discolored.

So, this starts the beginning of a new life for me, which I stayed undiagnosed for a long time.

The boy who stabbed me with the pencil received his "fill" from me on that first Monday we were in our new building. I waited patiently for him to arrive that morning. My friends entered inquiring how I was feeling at first, but my eyes were focused more on his arrival. Once he walked in, I grabbed him, even with all the pain I had, and I threw him across the room, tossing the new desks and chairs throughout the room. This event tore down the new blinds from the windows, and I continued to beat the living daylights out of him. Our homeroom teacher was the Principal who happened to hear the commotion and did our history teacher who resembled an NFL fullback bruiser who also came to pull us apart. Our parents were contacted, and we marched to the principal's office for the big "Why?" Today, I wish I could continue that story to have him eat the words "WHY!"

As the years proceeded, I continued to experience the lack of use of my right hand when I went to pick up a teacup or something intricate or if I did something like sewing. I continued to have spasms and distortion in my hand and pain in my arm, but it always seemed omitted and unnecessary by doctors to discuss during our visits. The burning pain, swelling, and I had the feelings of pins and needles remained a reminder that something was not right inside my arm and hand.

One evening when I went outside to put our pool ladder up for the night, and I turned around thinking it was in the locked position, only to discover that the ladder did not lock. The ladder had come crashing down onto the same arm that had been damaged by the pencil stabbing. We quickly made an appointment with the neurologist. With testing completed, we discovered that there was a tumor embedded in the upper portion of my right arm. At this juncture, the neurologist had diagnosed me with reflex sympathetic dystrophy (RSD), and the start of a laundry list of other medical concerns. Now, we are over 26-years of being misdiagnosed and will start a myriad of medications for various concerns. We are not even sure if any of this will help the cause. Plus, I started physical therapy for some type of strengthening and rebuilding in my arm and hand, and other treatments with the prognosis of healing completely. Unfortunately, none of this materializes.

I locate the RSDSA office only a few short miles from our home in New Jersey and I quickly became involved with their organization. I start reading more and more about RSD and I started to offer my help in any way that I could.

I also venture west to a doctor claiming he is working with RSD patients and is having extreme success in revitalizing these patients into "remission." This idea does not work either and as it turns out, this doctor ended up in prison for fraud.

Meanwhile, we are attempting acupuncture and other mediums until an article appears in the newspaper after further documentation was written about RSD, which reveals if you catch RSD within the first six months with treatment, medication, and physical therapy, you can put this into remission. Otherwise, you will end up in a wheelchair or worse for the rest of your life.

Well, forget that. I did not want to hear such news. Therefore, I started my support group in Burlington County, which developed into three support groups before I moved to Tennessee in 2006. We met regularly and even shared online discussions and telephone chats. So, when we moved, I made sure we would keep the word active in Tennessee as well as offering groups here.

The groups were open not only to the afflicted, but to their families and friends as this is where the support originates. With the Jersey groups, we would have fundraisers like our Afternoon of Elegance Tea Parties raising money to benefit RSDSA research and financial support for the afflicted. We would have local artists share their crafts via fashion shows, artwork, jewelry, where our guests could purchase from them at our teas and auctions. All proceeds, items sold, and monies made benefited the RSDSA 100%.

As the pain continued to worsen for me, I discovered Meilus Muscular Treatments to be helpful and then I came across Cold Laser Therapy and Fenzian Treatments which were beneficial to me that made a significant change in my life. I wrote several articles about this – one appearing in the RSDSA newsletter several years ago. These treatments have aided so many RSD patients and countless others. Where my cold and dark-colored limbs caused me so much pain, I would have these treatments, and the limbs would return to warm and normal pink color. The pain levels would decrease, and I would be a functional person for a while. I could even decrease some of my medication and perform tasks, unable to handle it before the treatments.

As the years have progressed, the RSD has spread throughout my body and into my internal organs. The latest is I am now in the third stage of kidney failure and watching my diet to hopefully stay away from dialysis. I have heart, lung, and blood clot issues and as I said earlier, a laundry list of other medical concerns.

My supportive, loving, and caring family stands by me completely during this ordeal. My husband is my steady rock and has been faithfully by my side throughout our entire relationship. We shall be married 50-years come 2020 and I thank God for him daily. To endure this monster and me, this long, he is a Saint for sure! It is a blessing for me to be surrounded by such wonderful children and family members who are always there to aid me through these most difficult times.

I hold firm to my faith, for without God in my life I doubt very much if I would be here today. For without Him, I am sure I would have taken a different path. He continues to bless me in so many different ways, saving my life many times sending the right people to me for that to be a reality. Even though I still am in pain and still have this affliction, He has been there to comfort my way, giving me hope that through Him all things are possible.

This affliction is quite suicidal, and I have lost many friends already. I have caught a few friends and acquaintances before succumbing to this, but it is getting tougher for people coping with the horrific pain that ravages our bodies from this culprit. People do not realize the anguish we bare daily as we "look too good to be ill and we must be faking it!" My answer has always been "Please come home with me. Spend the night in our home. See firsthand for yourself the life we lead. I guarantee you that you will not last six hours witnessing this pain should you decide to wear these shoes."

The one to 10 pain scale is antiquated – and thank goodness, they passed that prescriptions for medications to be scripted for chronic pain patients in the additional dosage amount that we require. I cut back on mine, so I could care for my Mother as her caregiver. It was tough to do; however, I wanted a clear mind to speak to the doctors and I just wanted to be the best, I could be for her, and I did NOT want to be involved with Pain Clinics that did absolutely NOTHING for me except to write a script for a couple of pills. They treated me like a piece of raw meat that caused enough feelings to eliminate any further visits to pain clinics and seek alternate ways to reduce my pain as I only needed just one small new script each month for a "few" pills. Given the third degree and placed through needless entry "lab work" and no help with psychological or knowledge of current aid for RSD, evoked enough interest to seek other sources of medical assistance for me.

I tried alternatives such as Akuamma, Kratom, and CBD oil. I have seen Brazilian healers, seen doctors across the country, taken every test in the book, and been involved with research studies. I hope and pray that one day soon I meet the person or persons that will face me and say, "we have the cure for RSD and we can correct the nerve that is damaged from this affliction!" I am throwing the biggest party ever and ALL of you are invited!

Sleepless nights full of pain – tossing and turning so much arrest, that even disturbs your soul mate's rest. Skin changes – peeling, discoloration, blotches and sores, swelling, pins & needles that turn into jostling stabs entering your body already consumed with enough fire that a fire extinguisher cannot filter your skin quickly enough to extinguish the enormous fire brewing internally.

The lack of social acceptance from the public, your friends, and even your family members, not realizing the severity of the extreme pain you are encountering through this ordeal, let alone realize the height of the pain levels this offers your system, leaving you to suffer on your own. The feel of sheets and blankets on our beds that are excessively hard and heavy for us to situate on our bodies and the need for them to be elevated by some type of contraption so they do not touch our skin as it sends our system into a destructive electronic storm. The feel of touch, hot or cold, as we shower, swim, or eat, sends us into a galaxy of raging electrified hornets. Even a simple hug or soft kiss can set our nervous system to a painful catastrophe. We devise ways to re-communicate with our soul mate to keep that sweet intimacy alive as long as we have a strong support system with them, as we need all their love to carry us forward.

The preface encouraging faithful indulgence into our daily homework, keeping abreast of the latest information on RSD-CRPS; and, then, in turn, offering all this information to our family, friends, doctors, and the public remains a true necessity on our behalf. We need to locate more medical people to come forward to our aid as the more awareness – the closer we are to that long-awaited miracle cure for us. Support groups are quite beneficial as we have the opportunity to not only meet other afflicted, but also share and learn more about our disease. We can share relaxation/focus imagery techniques and be a comfort to one another.

As long as there is a sun that rises every morning, there is a ray of hope for all of us. Hold strongly to this, hold fast to whatever faith you possess, pray – this does work, keep that beautiful, radiant smile upon our faces and we shall be the VICTORS! This monster will take a hike, I am confident of this. The cure is close – I am confident of this; and we shall survive the black fire hole we are presently in and truly be the winners of this amazing fight – TOGETHER – with Faith, Hope, and Prayers! God bless you all!

COMPLEX REGIONAL PAIN SYNDROME (CRPS): MY PERSONAL HELL
By: Tammy Parish

Hi, my name is Tammy, and I have suffered from CRPS for five years. I am 51-years old. I have three grown children and one amazing stepson who is 15-years old. For a long time, I was a single mom. I was raised in New Brunswick, Canada, but lived most of my adult life in the USA. I was married to an Air Force serviceman. We moved all over. (I divorced him years ago). In 2011, my kids and I moved from San Antonio, Texas to Barrie, Ontario. In 2013, I met my soulmate. Without his love and support, I probably wouldn't be here to tell my story. He takes me to 99% of my appointments. He listens to the doctors, as I never remember 10% of conversations. He helps me understand the things they say. He keeps me positive, picks up my prescriptions, he lets me cry on his shoulders, and he never complains at all. He goes to chronic pain classes with me. He helps me with everything, he accepts my limits and has had to take on so much more responsibility not only in our home but the finances too. We went from a dual-income home to a single income home; he now has to do all the driving if it's more than 30-minutes. He does not make me feel bad about the restrictions related to my disease. He didn't get upset when I missed his 50th birthday because of the meds I was on then made me a monster. He keeps the kids informed and updates them on everything. He is my everything! Our kids have had to do things children should not have to do at ages 11, 17, and 19. My daughters have had to not only dress me, but they also bathed me and have helped me in and out of bed. They have listened to me cry and have had to deal with many mood swings! My stepson has understood the many times I had to cancel on him. My daughter understood when I had to leave her high school graduation ceremony. You can't imagine how much I cried then. My only goal in life was seeing my children graduate high school!

138

That too was taken away from me. My stepson graduated from 8th grade and he was so looking forward to having us there, he was so excited to see us in the crowd. I could see his sad face when I had to get up and I slowly walked out. I laid in screaming pain in the back seat of our truck, just so my husband could see his son graduate.

I was an outgoing, outspoken person. I loved having fun, I was usually the life of the party. I love music and my passion was dancing. I loved to dance. My kids and I listened to music all the time. We would dance around the house all the time. I was very adventurous and loved trying out new things and I loved traveling.

On, October 14, 2014, I was rear-ended by a distracted driver. I was heading home from work; I was approaching a traffic light. As I was slowing down, I glanced into my rear-view mirror and noticed a red car was coming way too fast and I braced because I knew he was going to hit me. The night of the incident I had a bad headache (I normally didn't get headaches). I assumed it was just the drama of being hit and the stress of it all, as I only had my new car for a few months. The car accident was not too bad. He hit me at about 35-km.

The next day I went to work and had terrible neck and shoulder pain. Then I noticed my groin was hurting. Like something was caught or pulling and I was getting these weird electrical shocks from my groin up the side of my back and into the back of the right side of my head. Within the first few days, I saw my family doctor (I had three different ones since they were useless). I was prescribed muscle relaxants. The pain got worse and I continued to work, missing quite a few days going to physical therapy, massage therapy and doctor appointments, trying to figure out what was causing so much pain in my neck, shoulder, groin, and butt. I was sent to several different orthopedic surgeons and specialists for well over a year. I was told I needed a total hip replacement.

Then, I was told I didn't need a hip replacement. They saw bone spurs and an acetabular impingement.

I tried my best to continue to work while I was trying to find help for my pain. Going from doctor to doctor and therapy after therapy.

In, August of 2015, our HR girl and my immediate supervisor took me into the board room and said that I had missed 17-days so far and that if I missed another day, I would be fired. That afternoon, I had a doctor's appointment and told her, and she said she thought it was best if I went on short term disability. So, that is what I did.

By the time I stopped working, even now. I have not stopped trying to get help with this insane pain.

In, November of 2015, I had to have a hysterectomy due to ongoing female issues I had been having for some time after having an IUD.

In, March of 2016, one of the orthopedic surgeons that originally said I did not need a hip replacement did end up doing it. He felt that it would stop the ongoing pain. I was up for anything! I want the pain to stop!

At the six-week mark, I started physical therapy again. From the time I had the car accident until even now, I'm still looking for help with this damn pain!! Still working with yet another physical therapist. While doing physio I noticed the pain was by far worse than before the hip replacement. I would cry to my physiotherapist telling him that now my leg is in constant screaming pain and I mean CONSTANT! He suggested I needed "stronger pain medication" and that I had "pissed off, the muscles." He said that I needed to "push through the pain."

This pain differed from before the hip replacement. Now my right leg is constantly screaming in pain. It feels like my leg is on fire! It also feels like a bear claw is tearing up my muscles and nerves. At times, my leg feels like it's a hundred pounds. I constantly feel pulling, itchy, ripping, and burning from the front of my leg to my butt. My sacroiliac joint (SI joint) on the right side feels like a horse kicked me and my SI joint got stuck. My Piriformis is always throbbing, pulling, moving, and it feels like something is gnawing at it.

My ribs on my right side feel like they are bruised, and my neck and shoulder are always tight. My jaw pulls on the right side and at times it causes me to feel like I have an earache.

It even affects my collar bone. My occipital nerve feels so much pressure, it makes it tough to think. I get random electric shocks and muscle spasms. It feels like I am being shocked by a Taser. That's what it feels like. I have brain fog several times a day. My memory and cognitive skills are suffering. My toes spasm and I get feelings of pins and needles in my right foot. My joints ache and I get stiff if I stay in the same position for too long.

I get exhausted, extremely fast. If my leg gets touched, it sends signals to my brain telling me that the nerve endings are firing up. If I use my right arm too much, my brain goes crazy with too much pressure and my brain goes to crap. I don't have many dreams anymore because my brain is too focused on the pain. At times my head feels like it's been dropped on cement a few times. It's TERRIBLE!!

So, I tried many different medications...Lyrica, Cymbalta, hydromorphone, tramadol, lidocaine infusions, lorazepam, gabapentin, nabilone, butran (buprenorphine) patches. The list is endless, not to mention the horrible side effects of these drugs and having to take more medications to counteract these medications.

Issues with constipation, intense sweats, dry mouth, hemorrhoids, brain fog, zombie-like feelings, vomiting, night terrors, insomnia, mood swings. The list is endless. My days are spent lying on a heating pad, pacing, hot Epsom salt baths, meditations, stretching, self-talk, Yoga,

141

mindfulness and trying to educate myself on CRPS. Going to the hospital is useless. They don't know or understand CRPS. They treat you like you are mentally unstable!

Three times I had to go to the ER because I could not stop the spasms and the pain was unbearable. All three times, I ended up going home and medicating myself as much as possible just to get through it.

I was told I had SI joint dysfunction, Piriformis syndrome, myofascial pain, musculoskeletal pain, degenerative disc disease (DDD), trochanteric bursitis, soft tissue injury of the cervical spine and iliopsoas bursitis and CRPS.

My journey has been long and tough. Not only have I had to deal with terrible doctors that are paid off by the insurance companies. I also have to now deal with depression and anxiety. We are told so many different things. Use ice. Don't use ice. Rest the leg, keep the leg moving, use a cane, don't use a cane, journal, don't journal... it's endless.

While trying to figure out where all this insane screaming pain is coming from, I had to deal with the lawsuit. I find it funny that I went through a total hip replacement, been on every medication possible, tried every therapy possible and yet doctors are paid to say there is nothing wrong.

So, the massage therapist, physiotherapy, yoga therapy, pool therapy, naturopathic therapy, mindfulness, cognitive-behavioral therapy (CBT), spiritual healing, meditation, acupuncture, IMS, cortisone injections, Synvisc injections, medical marijuana, CBD oil, ketamine infusion, is this all for nothing? Are all these people injecting me, poking me, medicating me... all for their benefit? I have done everything imaginable, even paid out of my pocket to go to Buffalo, NY to figure out what is happening.

The doctor in Buffalo ensured me that it was not in my head. He did a Tenjet procedure that showed the tendons are "grossly hypoechoic" and thickened with loss of fibrillar echotexture. The greater Trochanteric showed cortical remodeling and spur formation consistent with enthesopathy.

Doctors who were paid by the insurance companies say that I made it up in my head, that I'm looking for "a pay out." Lol! Who in their right mind would go through everything I have gone through? I have done everything you can imagine getting help. Pay out of pocket with no job. I don't understand why doctors are paid to write false reports discrediting a person who lives in severe pain. I fight hard enough every single minute, to fight the constant screaming in my leg.

I have been lucky enough to have finally found a good family doctor, she does not know much about CRPS, but she is always there for me.

Living with CRPS has been just unexplainable. I can tell you until the cows come home, how much pain my leg is in and you would find it hard to believe. I FIND IT HARD TO BELIEVE! I cannot wrap my head around the fact that I will live like this forever? I will continue to have to medicate myself daily and continue with trials of things to help, all still wondering what they are doing to my body. CRPS has changed my life by a 100%! I can't focus like I used to, I can't enjoy things like I used to because the pain is so loud that it is ALWAYS FIRST, THE PAIN IS ALWAYS FIRST!! I used to play cards, go on vacation and do excursions, drive across the country (now I drive 30-minutes or less), I used to love to dance, can't do that, swimming in the ocean used to be easy, now I can barely walk into the ocean, the waves are just too much! I can't do any winter activities, gardening, amusement parks are out now, no jumping of any sort, I can't enjoy a girl's weekend like I used to, now... I have to plan everything I do. If I want to go, see a movie. I have to do NOTHING all day long just so I can sit through it, not to mention I have to take extra meds on days I go out. Even watching TV or listening to music can be difficult because your pain keeps your focus. I used to dress up every year for Halloween, it was one of my favorite holidays. I'd go dancing all night long.

Sex, I can no longer enjoy my husband, and it takes everything! Thinking, concentration, escaping the pain, and trying to relax. You just can't relax enough to enjoy intimacy.

CRPS has changed how I interact with people. When my pain is high, it is difficult to concentrate. I have to cancel plans, I stay behind. They see me cry and don't know what to say or do. People get tired of hearing, you complain constantly. They simply can't understand.

I was a single mom of three amazing children. My focus and priority, was to raise them. I thought that once they were all out of high school, then my job was done, and I could focus on me. Ha-ha... Was I wrong?

I now spend my days just getting through them one day at a time. There are days when I can't even get out of bed. Those days, I try to use more mindfulness and meditation. When you are in severe pain, your mind tends to go very dark. Now that I have had four Ketamine infusions, I'm not suicidal as much. So far, ketamine infusions have been the only thing to tone down the screaming pain a bit. I have almost given up a few times it has come to close.

When you plan it and have it all worked out, that is too close! I would have never even thought of suicide before all this. Now it's part of this and I have to fight it!! Not a single doctor out there cared if I took my life!

My moods can be so deep, it scares me. I have to fight this war continuously.

I have journaled some of my days, writing about the pain, wishing it would stop. Some doctors say to write a journal, others say journaling only keeps you in the pain. So, sometimes I do, sometimes I don't.

I have been treated so poorly by nurses who had never even heard of CRPS. I had to contact the hospital to make a complaint about how I was treated. Living with CRPS makes you feel exhausted quickly, from doing the smallest things in life. Your mood depends on the pain level. Let's be honest here, the pain scale cannot be used for CRPS patients. The pain is so far off, that when I say it's a "4" today, it's a "4" that normal people would never imagine.

The pain of CRPS is real and is not in my mind! I live in horrible pain every second of the day!

In summary, I was fine before this car accident. I would not have needed a total hip replacement at the young age of 48. Since the hip replacement, I have been in severe pain, causing depression and anxiety. I feel lost and confused most often. I have learned a lot about the ignorance of the medical community and how I thought that all doctors took an oath to help those in need. I learned that money is worth more than life to some. I learned that you have to fight for yourself because no one else will. I'm learning not to give up.

CRPS is Hell! A private hell! It can't be completely explained. Because I look "good," and I have a few (what looks like to others) decent moments, that people don't believe I'm in this much pain daily. You have to smile as to not offend those who are tired of listening to you. You find out who your true friends are! You find out the family members who truly care and those who think you are full of crap and believe you made it all up for attention. Lol! Attention! Who goes through all this for attention?

I understand why they call this the suicide disease. Try living in constant chronic pain, nothing stops it, nothing helps it, there are no breaks from it and worst of all... no one sees it. I'm sorry for all the families who have lost a loved one to this horrific disease, but I promise you, they are no longer suffering in a silent hell. For those of us making it through another day, we show strength, courage, self-worth, and fight. Keep fighting, keep looking for help, keep the conversation going. We just might save a life.

A side-note from my big sister

Well, my sister, Tammy was asked to write about her CRPS. It's about being a Guinea pig and experiment for drugs and compiling of doctors who want to help but don't even understand or know what CRPS is.

My name is Tina and I am Tammy's older sister. We grew up healthy, in a family of six girls who never missed Christmas, birthdays and events that were truly in our hearts because the family was our most important thing in life. Not anymore! CRPS has changed the dynamics of our family, and we don't blame Tammy, but we do blame CRPS.

I am crying as I write this because I want my sister to forgive me for not understanding CRPS. I live 12-hours away from Tammy and when she would call me complaining and crying about her disease, I truly did not know the severity of it. Until... I recently lived with her this past July and August. I got to see first-hand the excruciating painful life my little sister has to endure, every moment of every day. CRPS consumes her like a black cloak, a demon that sucks the happy right out of my sister. Her days are trying hard to get out of bed with a smile for me. I can see her pale face twitch from trying to sleep at night. I can hear her up during the night crying. When my sister sits next to me in a chair with her leg up on an ottoman, I can see the muscle spasms in her toes as we crochet together. I can hear her deep breathing from the pain shooting through her and the jolts her whole body does as she tries to cope. We go for groceries and we have to stop until she repositions herself. Tammy has to bring her cane with her, meds, extra supplies with her just in case something happens unexpectedly this is all takes up precious time.

Tammy is strong, but for four years now she is still fighting to get help.

She struggles with traumatic emotions. Those emotions are extensions of the chronic pain that attack her randomly all day long and all night long. I cannot imagine being shocked, jolted, burning pain, acute brain pain, nerves jumping around randomly from head to toe, headaches, blackouts, the pressure on her joints and muscles. She complains about this and I'm sure I have not remembered all of her complaints. Please, if you read this, I want others to know that if your loved one says "it hurts," believe them! Support them! You can keep telling them to try to push forward for themselves and listen because it's important to them.

I will do whatever it takes to support my little sister and listen to her complain, any minute of every day because I want her with my family and her family for as long as possible.

Sincerely, a sister who has witnessed CRPS and knows it's a devastating disease that debilitates her body, stresses her mind and traumatizes her emotions. I have witnessed this brutal attack on my sister Tammy. I hope and pray this helps others understand the pain from this horrible disease. Love, Tina

MY CRPS STORY
By: Jacqueline Neff

In 1994, I was in the Army. While running, I sustained a soft tissue injury to my left knee. The pain kept getting worse, so they discharged me. I came home and was awarded a 10% disability, but was told that I had tendonitis. The pain kept getting worse over the years and spread to my right leg. The doctors kept telling me it was all in my head or treated me like I was faking it.

In 2015, I was desperate, as my condition had progressed so much that I was having problems functioning, and my depression had got the best of me. I went to an orthopedic specialist the VA referred me to, and he did more tests and said, he couldn't find anything wrong. The VA canceled any further visits. I went into the VA and demanded to go back to the Ortho. This time, they sent me to the Chillicothe, Ohio, VA Medical Center Orthopedic Department. When the doctor was about to test my knee reflexes, I burst into tears and begged her not to. She said she'd only seen that one other time and referred me to pain management there. That's when I was finally diagnosed with complex regional pain syndrome (CRPS).

She said that my condition had progressed so far that the only thing she felt would help was a spinal cord stimulator (SCS). I was referred to a local pain management center to have the implant done. For five glorious months, I was pain-free. Then, it simply stopped helping. I had it adjusted with no results. The pain was worse than before, had spread to everywhere from the waist down, and my spine now burned horribly. I simply shut it off and sought more help. I've been on many medications, but nothing has helped, and some made me so sick I couldn't take it long enough to see if it would help.

I've been to several pain management doctors with no results or help with treating my pain. I had to fire my old primary care doctor at the VA because she yelled at me and called me a pill seeking faker. I am currently not taking medications, and it has spread internally and to both upper arms and it sometimes affects my hands. I've been fighting with the VA for several years, trying to get a rate increase. I'm on social security.

I spend most of my time in bed because most days I can barely walk to the bathroom. This disease has destroyed my life and I don't even care that I'm alive hardly anymore. My depression and anxiety, has been off the charts. I'm lonely because I've lost so many friends who just don't understand. My husband, Scott, is great though. He sees my pain. He sees me struggling to try simple things and goes out of his way to take care of me even though he works 16-hours a day five to six days a week. It's not fair to him to have to work so hard then have to take care of dinner, the house, the pets and me. I feel like such a burden. I used to hike, fish, camp and loved being outside. Now I can't do any of it. I'm lost.

I hope my story helps other patients.

BOBBY'S RSD STORY
By: R.S.

I had a good job, a wonderful wife (Susan) and we loved to travel. I was a marathon runner and hiker.

In 2010, the life I had known had abruptly changed.

In September of 2010, I fell and broke my left calcaneus. I went to a prominent foot and ankle surgeon in Philadelphia who kept me in a cam boot for seven months. I explained to this doctor that I didn't think it was normal for my foot to burn fiercely, but he didn't believe me.

And so, the journey began...

I made an appointment with a doctor at the Rothman Institute after I received an electrical shock in my foot akin to putting my hand into an electrical socket. He said it could be reflex sympathetic dystrophy (RSD) but he hoped it was not. I made an appointment with Doctor R.S., who was the "RSD guru" and had a three-year wait to see him. Six months, before my appointment, he retired.

I made another appointment with another doctor at Hahnemann who understood RSD and the wait was a year. Two weeks, before my appointment they called and said the doctor had personal problems and was not seeing patients any longer. We found out that he went to jail for sexual abuse.

Finally, I was diagnosed by Doctor R.S.'s., replacement as having RSD.

My wife Susan fought to have me enrolled in a clinical trial at Hahnemann for plasmapheresis. After seven months of back and forth, we were accepted. It was a nightmare as the left hand did not know what the right hand was doing. After the port was placed in my chest, and I had a couple of treatments, we left. It seemed dangerous to be in a trial that was so, disorganized and our questions were met with puzzled faces.

I went to a neurologist who put me on Nucynta for years. He charged $1500 for the first appointment and $500 each month only to spend five minutes with me and give me a script.

I continued to search out doctors because they did not believe me when I described my symptoms and said that there was no such thing as RSD. I found a pain doctor who put me on MS Contin 30 mg ER and 30 mg, IR as the Nucynta was not working as it had been. I tried nerve blocks four times and ketamine once without positive results.

I developed RSD in my eyes and became photosensitive, so I had to wear sunglasses in the house.

I felt like I had a piece of glass in my eyes for two years. I went to six Ophthalmologists, and all six doctors did not understand my pain. They all said it was dry eye.

Finally, I found a doctor in Boston who did believe me, but nothing could be done for the searing burning eye pain. I am grateful that it went into remission after two years.

I developed back issues which include advanced degenerative disk disease, bulging disks, severe right and left neural foraminal stenosis, compression of L-5 nerve roots and pars fracture bilateral.

Six doctors, including the Hospital for Special Surgery said I need spinal fusion surgery. I said that I am not doing this surgery!

I tried acupuncture, but the pain from the needles in my back sent me to the ER as the pain was unrelenting. They found nothing other than the back issues listed above and were puzzled as to why the acupuncture would have caused this level of pain.

I was going to a pool so that I could walk back and forth to gain strength and increase my mobility. I enjoyed it and went daily. Unfortunately, someone defecated in the pool and it was closed for a couple of days.

I went back to the pool as soon as it reopened, and had the same electric shock, I got in my foot, but this time it was in my penis. The burning pain followed and it was awful. I went to see a few urologists, and again I was not believed. One doctor put me on Cipro for a month (a no-no for RSD patients) and then I was put on another antibiotic for months. I found nothing helped and I was no longer going to the pool.

I was having shortness of breath and coughing and as my wife signed me up to see a concierge doctor, she called him and asked for a CT scan of the chest. The pulmonologist said I had a rather large hiatal hernia and severe asthma and prescribed a high dose of steroids. I had bad side effects, so my wife called and I began to titrate quicker than was initially prescribed, but she got the ok from the nurse.

After two days on the steroids, I was told that my wife couldn't wake me up, so she called 911 and they took me to the ER. I was unable to verbalize properly and was talking gibberish. I tried to remove the IV. They did every possible test and proceeded to take me off of all of my psychiatric meds. They put me in restraints, and I fell off of the bed as they had left me with one restraint on. I hurt myself and at that point, I could not urinate.

That is when they inserted a Foley Cath. Which I have to this day. With RSD in my penis!

My behavior was way out of whack. It was like I was psychotic, and I was moved to a nursing home. No one understood what was going on and I was "out of my mind." It lasted for over a month and it turns out that I was suffering from a psychotic episode due to the steroids.

This is not an uncommon occurrence and finally, when we did research, we found it to be the answer to my bizarre behavior.

A concierge doctor should care for the patient whenever he is needed. This doctor told me that I was taking up too much of his time, and he had to move on with other patients. He did not call when I was in the hospital or the nursing home. Susan spent eight hours a day at the nursing home and continued to be my fierce advocate. She caught many mistakes by the nurses and aides and finally took me home.

Susan found a new concierge doctor who was compassionate and a great diagnostician.

I wanted to know why I could not urinate, but the urologist said, I should go see a neurosurgeon and vice versa. I visited a neurosurgeon who said I should go to the hospital as he said I didn't seem right and with weakness in my legs and had a Cath, I should have more testing. The team found nothing. They wanted me to have EMG.

They sent me to a new urologist where they did urodynamic testing. It was painful. He suggested cystoscopy and suprapubic Cath. I am not a candidate for the Suprapubic Cath as the back pain and vertebrae pushing me forward along with the burning RSD in my penis would preclude the placement of the tube. Both procedures are invasive and as with all invasive procedures, may create a new pain generator (as the EMG did).

My new concierge doctor sent me to another neurologist who ordered an EMG which I wish I never had, as it caused excruciating pain in L-5 and down to my buttocks. The only conclusion was that I did not have neuropathy. Nothing else!

If I could only sleep!!! I can only sleep a couple of hours at a time and am woken up by the pain. That is with a sleeping pill.

I am grateful for the unconditional love that Susan has for me as well as being a fierce advocate for my care. We have been together for 30-years and love each other.

She has devoted her life to me, and I wish I could be a more active participant in our relationship, but we will never give up in the fight against this vicious, ugly disease.

COMPLEX REGIONAL PAIN SYNDROME (CRPS): A LIFE SENTENCE
By: Lizbeth Rice

My name is Lizbeth Rice and I've been living with complex regional pain syndrome (CRPS) for over 20-years now. I developed it from surgery. I had arthritis in my left foot from a terrible break from years prior. The podiatrist who did the surgery was going to fuse the bones with screws. After the surgery, my pain was worse. My foot was bright red, and I had burning pain. The doctor told me that I was simply healing. After walking around on it for a year, the pain was worse. I knew something was wrong. My insurance company didn't want me to go to an orthopedic surgeon. I could see the top of one of the screws coming up from my foot. After fighting, the insurance company, I was able to see an orthopedic surgeon. He had to do a new surgery to remove the screw. He told me that there was a large screw holding down tendons and it had severed a large nerve. He had to fuse other bones that hadn't been done and remove the screws that were not put in correctly.

I was told that nothing more could be done, and I continued to work to raise my daughter. I was in constant pain. In 2002 I saw another doctor and he told me that I had CRPS. I didn't understand the name and assumed that he was just saying that I was in pain. I continued to see other doctors. I found one doctor that told me it was called reflex sympathetic dystrophy (RSD). I looked it up and I finally realized what it was. I was then able to know what I was dealing with. I had six nerve blocks, and they didn't work. I then had a spinal cord stimulator (SCS) implant. It was a nightmare. The leads kept moving and I had to have surgeries to change the batteries. After about four years I had it removed. They left the wires in because they said I had too much scar tissue.

I got to the point that I couldn't work anymore and that has been a big strain on me financially. I had to go on Social Security. I can barely afford to pay my rent, pay bills and buy food. I have been off work since 2005. I've lost all my friends. I can't do anything anymore. I am on pain medication to get by. I barely leave my house and I am mostly confined to the couch or bed. The CRPS has spread to my waist down. I have terrible back problems from the SCS. I have grandkids and they're what's keeping me alive.

This is a horrible disease that has ruined my life. I have been very depressed. But I have learned that this is the way it will be for the rest of my life. I am 58-years old and I have a life sentence for something that I don't deserve.

LIVING WITH CRPS
By: Sharon Shepherd

Hi, my name is Sharon Shepherd and I live in Melbourne, Australia. On the 18th of May 2009, I was at work doing my normal duties when my foot became stuck to the floor, and I had no idea why. All the guys in the factory were standing around and laughing at me because I was stuck to the floor, so with everything I had I ripped my foot up and realized the guys had put glue on the floor as a practical joke, thank God it was almost time to go home as I was in pain. When I got home, I took my steel cap boots off, it simply swelled up like crazy, and I could hardly walk. The next day, I got up and my foot was still swollen so I went to the doctors and he put me on crutches and then my daughter-in-law took me to work so I could report what happened to me and give them my certificate. Well, I have been off work for two weeks now and I'm still in pain and I'm off the crutches.

Well, I am going shopping with my niece and we are going down an escalator that wasn't working when my knee gave way and I fell so off to the doctors again, my General Practitioner (GP) put me straight back on the crutches again. After about two months and still, in pain he said he was sure I had nerve damage and said it was called reflex sympathetic dystrophy (RSD) which I had no idea what that was. My GP gave me an information sheet to read up on it and referred me to a pain specialist. As we all know your very first appointment is to tell them what your problem is and how it happened. So, after a few visits and medication, I went back to work on modified duties and hours as I was still on my crutches and could only put Ugg boots on so I worked in the office a couple of days a week and a couple of hours a day.

I did get back out on the floor in the warehouse still with my Ugg boots on as the swelling has not gone down so I'm still doing modified hours and sitting and standing until one day I was coming out of the bathroom when one of the guys said to another Sharon must of got f##ked up the arse last night look at how she walks and that's because my foot turned so much that my ankle almost hitting the ground. When my daughter-in-law picked me up from work as I couldn't drive, I asked her to take me straight to the doctors as I was hurting and from that day in September 2008 on, I never went back.

Since leaving work I have felt lost as I loved my job, but that day in May 2008, changed my life for the worst. It's really hard to get around as I can't drive so I was relying on my son and his girlfriend to get me to all my appointments and the amount, of doctors I have seen is crazy, but I feel like I'm broken and can't be fixed. There has been a lot of crying because the pain would get so bad, I couldn't sleep just having a doona (quilt) on my foot was hell.

As the years have passed and I have lost a lot of friends because you say yes to going out and when the time comes to do it you can't because of the pain. I understand how people would get sick of it canceling all the time. At about one and a half years after my accident, I had to have driving lessons in a car with a left foot accelerator as I can't drive with my right foot. I had about six driving lessons with the left foot and it was hard at first, but I got it, now I don't think I could ever drive with my right foot again.

It's been over ten years since my accident and I'm still in a lot of pain. I still see a pain specialist as my spinal cord stimulator (SCS) is not working as it should be. Fifteen out of the 32 electrodes were not working, so they said, I will have to have these removed and have new ones put in. I'm a bit scared because after the first ones were put in, I had to go back into surgery in August as my back got infected five months after the surgery. I still take Gabapentin 900 mg three times a day to help with the pain and can have up to six Endone (Oxycodone) per day.

Since this has happened, I now also have depression, which I take Endep (Amitriptyline) for. Every day is different some days are good, some are bad, it also depends on the weather when it's hot my foot swells up so much it's hard to walk for very long and to find shoes that will fit. When it's cold the pain almost doubles and can still swell, in the winter too, so I can't win either way.

Treatments
Used underarm crutches from May 2009 for about 12 months.
From about 11/6/2009 till 12/10/2009 I had 37 sessions of physiotherapy.
In December 2009 I had an ultrasound guided right Hallux sesamoid injection.
Sympathetic lumbar infusion from 08/11/2010 till 12/11/2010.
Epidural infusion 28/02/2011 till 05/03/2011
Cam boot from May 2010 till November 2011.
Ketamine infusion from the 16/11/2011 till 13/12/2011.
Trial of spinal cord stimulator from 10/10/2012 till 31/10/2012.

CRPS FOLLOWING A KNEE REPLACEMENT
By: E.R.

I developed complex regional pain syndrome (CRPS) following a knee replacement in June 2018. For a while, my progress was normal, but after about four weeks I struggled to walk. My follow up appointment with the surgeon was brought forward, and I was admitted to a rehabilitation hospital for two weeks, where I was told that I needed to wear compression stockings all the time, as blood wasn't circulating properly back to my brain. I was put on several different types of walking frames (pick up, 2-wheel, 4-wheel) and eventually crutches, and sent home. Part of the problem was psychological, I was told.

Every time I visited the surgeon, and he looked at my swollen, shiny, cold, blue leg, he would first ask about my pain levels. (This was because he suspected CRPS, but as my pain levels weren't over the top, I couldn't have it, was the reasoning.) He was more concerned that I wasn't walking well and had less than 90-degree bend.

Once able to do hydrotherapy I started at my local pool, where an excellent physiotherapist helped me to become more confident in the water and do an increasingly difficult program of exercises as my abilities improved. However, when she first saw me, she was horrified. I was the most difficult case she had seen in many years of practice. She told me that I had either had a stroke or had CRPS. I had never heard of the latter, but went to my GP, who was happy to organize an MRI which showed no stroke. It took another few months before he was happy to refer me to a pain specialist.

The pain specialist was interesting. I don't have allodynia, but have all the other symptoms of CRPS, so he diagnosed 'Atypical CRPS'. Apart from referring me to a Rehabilitation Centre, and telling me, he wants to give me a nerve block, I haven't found him helpful. The Cochrane Library tells me that I have a 10% chance of getting Neuralgia if I have the nerve block.

Given the probability of getting CRPS from a knee replacement is much smaller than that, I'm not happy with proceeding. I will only do so if I stop improving with the other treatment.

Symptoms: swollen, shiny, very cold, blue leg, particularly my big toe; nerve pain, which increases during the day. This I describe as being between having all the hairs on my leg stand on end, and pins and needles; a bit like having thousands of insects crawling under my skin all at the same time. Every morning when I wake up, I am usually pain-free. As soon as I get out of bed and put weight on my leg, I can have a huge range of different pains. 1. The original injury, a torn cartilage from 1971, 2. Post-surgery pain, 3. Pre-surgery osteoarthritis pain 4. Nerve pain. Occasionally I get the normal flare pain, of the feeling of burnt knives cutting through my flesh. This doesn't last longer than a day. I still have difficulty walking. Once in walking mode, which can take several seconds to initiate, I have difficulty in stopping unexpectedly or changing directions. If I do stop, I stand still for quite a while, trying to get into walking mode again.

I used to use a walking stick, but have returned to using a single crutch because I've found that strangers are better at keeping their distance when they see a woman with a crutch rather than a woman with a walking stick. People used to walk straight through me and still do sometimes. It's not uncommon for my stick to be completely pushed out from underneath me. Just as well, I'm doing lots of balance exercises in the pool.

The scariest symptom is also the most bizarre. Sometimes when I go to walk, a voice in my head yells out to me "Stop! Remember, you don't have a left leg!" But I do. (Almost phantom limb syndrome, but with the limb still attached)

Treatment? Apart from the post-surgery pain killers for about six weeks, I have taken no medication. Panadol didn't make any difference, and I can cope mostly with the pain, which is mostly nerve pain.

Hydrotherapy has been good when the pool is warm enough. I am now much stronger than before and have excellent balance. At the Rehabilitation Centre (starting in February 2019) I have been seeing an Occupational therapist (two sessions earlier this year), a psychologist (about five sessions earlier this year), and a physiotherapist (weekly sessions for about six months then fortnightly for a couple of months, and monthly at the moment).

Physiotherapy has been interesting. First, I used cards showing pictures of knees from all angles to be able to determine the left and right knees as quickly as possible. (40 cards in well under a minute). Then I did many months of mirror therapy (covering my bad leg and moving my good leg in front of a mirror.) About two months ago, while exercising in front of the mirror, a little voice in my head said, "Look at your left leg go!" I was using my right leg. I've have been recently told that I don't need to do any more of this.

I have had a few minutes when my brain fog lifts and my leg feels normal and I walk without any aids, but that's three occasions since January. I've probably walked a total of 50-meters without aids since surgery.

How has CRPS changed my life? For some time, I wasn't welcome at my son and daughter-in-law's house. I was told I was lazy, unhelpful, not wanted (but your husband is very welcome!) This caused deep distress as I loved my grandchildren dearly. They were the most positive reason to live, and if the ban had extended, I doubt I'd be here now. I became quite depressed. More recently I have been welcome. I suspect in part the problem was due to post-natal depression (not mine). When there I tend to sit in the same chair – it's the only one that I find it easy to get out of and play with the grandchildren. As I've improved, I've been able to cook meals and help with caring for the children (aged 1 and 3), but there's a lot I can't do, such as lift them unless I'm seated. My house is dirty (husband vacuums every six months or so), I've recently found someone to help with the gardening (I used to call my backyard my edible jungle, as we'd eat something from there every meal).

I miss gardening. (I couldn't get down, therefore many months until the rails were put by the steps and wire put on the steps to stop them being slippery.)

It took six months before I realized that I should get a disabled parking permit (November 2018). Getting this disabled parking permit has made it easier to travel around and get to places. Until then, I had been reliant on my husband to drive me everywhere. If we can get a parking space near where we want to go, it's great.

We've stopped doing many things we used to do, e.g., go to the cinema (I can't manage the stairs or escalators), football games (ditto), dancing (he goes without me), yoga, travel (I can't manage public transport, such as getting on/off trains which move on schedule rather than wait for a passenger to get her leg in walking mode), at a club dinner I had to sit downstairs while everyone else had their meal upstairs, my hair needs cutting, but I can't walk from the carpark to the salon, I need new glasses, etc.

What I'd like to see in public education is how to approach people using walking aids. I hate it when people walk straight through me, expecting me to get out of their way, even though I'm obviously using a crutch. I have trouble stopping. I have trouble changing directions. I have trouble starting to walk again when I have to stop. I hate it when my stick or crutch is pushed out from under me, as one of these days I may fall from being so unbalanced.

More about me: I tore my knee cartilage in a bad fall in 1971, when I was being stalked walking home from work, the third night in a row. At the time stalking wasn't an offense, and there were no mobile phones, no one to talk to about the problem. I had a meniscectomy in about 1974, as I wanted to have children, but kept falling over when my knee randomly gave way underneath me. I worked for the ABS. I had a drug free births of both my children, so I'm not a wimp when it comes to pain. Following the completion of receiving my B.Sc., I worked as a tutor and computer programmer then succumbed to tenosynovitis (swollen, cold, blue right arm, with pain worse than shingles and allodynia – sounds like CRPS to me, but I didn't understand that my pain level wasn't normal for tenosynovitis so didn't mention it to the doctor, in 1985, during the RSI epidemic. In Tasmania, one couldn't get the Worker's Compensation unless one had tenosynovitis.). I eventually recovered in the 1990s and retrained as a minister of religion. (Recovery this time: I used to meditate, had acupuncture and was taught how to use visualization to warm my hand).

I retired in 2015. Over time the pain in my knee became gradually worse, from osteoarthritis due to the lack of a gap between the bones in my knee. The idea of having surgery sounded good, but I decided that rather than wait until the pain was extreme, it would be better to have the surgery while I was younger to enable faster recovery.

Even though I was well screened before surgery, I didn't know that I was probably at risk for CRPS following the 1985 illness.

So, what went wrong? Where and when did my brain/parasympathetic nervous system lose my leg? My surgeon was very keen to have X-rays done on my knee, a few days after surgery. I was later told by the nurse that the X-rays had been returned. I asked if someone would explain them to me, but no one did. The following day I asked again, but still, no one did. The day after this I was given the X-rays to take home with me. The X-rays were eventually explained to me by the surgeon a couple of months later, but by then I had already lost my ability to walk.

I think my brain decided that because there were unanswered questions there was a problem with my leg, which took its own course of action as a result.

E.R.

Australia

"A WARRIOR'S SURVIVAL": SHANNON'S RSD STORY
By: Shannon Killebrew

Allow me to introduce myself, my name is Shannon Killebrew. I am using my full name as I have found that so many physicians, nurses, surgeons, and caregivers no longer see me as myself... They see a disease. I am still Shannon. I am still myself in spirit, even though reflex sympathetic dystrophy (RSD) has robbed me of almost all, but my heart beat.

All my life I seemed to have small oddities that were annoyances. From a child, I would wake in the night with agonizing leg pains. The pediatricians diagnosed me with "growing pains." The only relief was high doses of Tylenol and a warm, soaking bath in the middle of the night. As the years progressed, I had knee issues in High School and was diagnosed with subluxation of the patella. I had also discovered in middle school, I had severe scoliosis. To me, these issues were the norm and I adjusted accordingly.

I underwent several pelvic surgeries beginning at age 29 for various ovary issues. I noticed that after each surgery my legs and knees would be weak for months. My life seemed to make a comeback until one day in June when I was on my knees on a wooden bench trying to peer into a viewing room of the local Veterinary office to get a better look at kittens for adoption. My right knee twisted, and I had severe burning pain. I grimaced and it passed in a few minutes. Approximately one week afterward, I awoke from a sound sleep to the most agonizing pain in my right knee. I truly thought someone had broken into my home and stabbed me in my sleep! I expected blood-soaked sheets, but there was no injury. I began limping that day. I used an ace bandage and hobbled for approximately a week. The edema was worse by the day, as was the pain. Within weeks I brought out crutches from storage (from my high school days) and struggled as I had stairs in my home.

At this time, I had begun seeking answers. My PCP referred me to an orthopedist who immediately diagnosed the issue as a weak patella and ordered physical therapy. My knee was so swollen I could not wear pants and my feet were mottled a lovely bluish purple. I was so sensitive I only wore shorts. I could not tolerate socks or shoes. Physical therapy was out of the question. I was sent for X-rays, CT scans and eventually an MRI. All results were normal. I was then referred to a rheumatologist who was also confounded. Within six weeks I could no longer bear weight and a wheelchair was ordered by my orthopedist.

I continued the quest for answers. It was a grueling course of researching online, scheduling appointments, traveling...Which in itself was unbearable at times. I was blessed with a boyfriend who worked 12-hour shifts so he had three days off each week, which were spent traveling to appointments. I had so much imaging that I was forbidden any further X-rays for five years (radiation). I underwent so much serology that I developed scar tissue in my veins and became anemic. At one point a rheumatologist was desperate and placed me on a high dose prednisone regimen which caused severe depression and lifelong side effects (which I still suffer from to this day) including ocular hypertension and neuropathy.

During this time, I was determined to stay ambulatory, so I was still using crutches a good bit. I'd sit on my first stair step and use my arms to propel myself up & down the stairs. Within months, this issue was too difficult and my boyfriend would carry me down the stairs in the am and I would stay downstairs until bedtime when he would carry me back up. Those were terrifying trips as I had a steep staircase, and he could not see his feet! Within about ten months of using the crutches, I had caused such damage to my shoulders that I developed bilateral adhesive capsulitis (frozen shoulder... Both). I later discovered this was very common with RSD patients. I was then forced into a wheelchair permanently with the intermittent use of a scooter.

My home was not ADA accessible so a "not so lovely" portable toilet was brought in to sit in the living room for me as neither my wheelchair nor toilet would fit through my bathroom doorway. I was growing more hopeless by the minute. The pain, edema, and changes to my skin were horrible. I was also losing arm use and strength by the day.

I was so desperate that I found an orthopedic surgeon willing to do exploratory surgery hoping for an answer. The surgery revealed a full-thickness meniscus tear in my right knee (apparently from months before when my knee cap had twisted). I thought "Hallelujah, thank you, Lord, we found it, repaired it and now on with my life!" I adhered to the prescribed course of post-op care and physical therapy with only declining health and the pain level increasing. I eventually realized I had no choice but to move to a one-level home. In the process of trying to relocate my orthopedist decided surgery on my worst shoulder was now in order. I literally arranged a move of my home and physically relocated my wheelchair-bound self (pets included) into a small apartment and had surgery three days after the move! I did all of this with my right arm in a sling and while learning to use my left hand (I was right hand dominant). I was becoming mentally, physically and emotionally exhausted!!

At this point, I could walk a few steps from time to time. I moved, settled in and had my surgery over four days. I requested that the surgery center be very careful with my right leg as I still had no confirmed diagnosis. I suspected RSD. After the shoulder surgery, I never ambulated again. I awoke in recovery with significant jaw pain. I never chewed solid food after that surgery. My jaw was hyperextended for intubation and it caused the RSD to spread into my jaws, cheeks, and gums. The RSD then also mirrored to my left leg as well.

I was now non-ambulatory 100%, both legs affected, one arm in a sling recovering from surgery and I couldn't chew food.

I followed the protocol for post-op care, but never regained full use. I now focused on dentists, oral surgeons, and oral medicine specialists. I had no dental insurance, so I used most of my savings. There were never conclusive answers. I accepted this as my "new normal," and my life of mashed potatoes, yogurt, soup, smoothies, and boost high protein began.

My boyfriend was becoming distraught and exhausted. Our lives were nothing but doctor visits, tests, and trying to figure out how I could bathe, dress, travel, and eat. During this time, he nearly lost his job due to the absences from hospitalizations and visits. This was contributing to my feelings of frustration and hopelessness.

I continued to improve with the use of my left hand and researched more. At this point, I had been to physicians in my home town, surrounding cities and surrounding states. This was to include Emory in Atlanta, GA, and Mayo Clinic in Jacksonville, FL. We were both exhausted, in every way.

My Diagnosis

I found an orthopedist who specialized in joint disorders online. He was in a small town two and a half-hour away. By this time, traveling was almost unbearable. I would sit in the back seat so I could prop my bad leg up across the seat. Having it down for extended periods was intolerable. (Of note: I sold my car to purchase an older model car which was large and roomy to accommodate my legs). I scheduled an appointment. We were skeptical. My boyfriend risked his job and we prepared for the trip. His office was in a small town, Jesup, GA. It was a super tiny office with approximately seven chairs in the waiting room! There were trophy fish and trophy deer heads on the wall.

Very rural, but everyone was so kind. The staff was minimal and flabbergasted we had traveled so far to come to them. The office was so tiny that my wheelchair would barely fit through the doorways into the rooms.

The doctor stepped in and was very humble, personable and compassionate. He respected that I highly guarding my legs and was terrified for anyone to touch them. He examined visibly, no physical touching.

He confirmed immediately my suspicions and agreed more radiology was dangerous. I mentioned a test that I had researched, a "three-phase bone scan" which I had been told by Mayo Clinic and Emory University was no longer performed. He stated, "yes, it is, and I'm ordering the test ASAP!" He faxed the order to Memorial Medical Center in Savannah, GA. (One hour from me, three-hours from him). The day came and I underwent the travel and five-hour test, with a rest midway. The results were conclusive a week later... "Findings consistent with RSD." We had a definitive name for the beast!!!

I was immediately ordered a regimen of aquatic therapy, physical therapy, tens units, and anti-inflammatories. The only aquatic therapy center was an hour away with each session beginning at five minutes. This was grueling...More time off for my driver and helper, gas money and little benefit. We managed all 15-visits before insurance had a cap. The traditional physical therapy was touch therapy to acclimate me to touch and sensation. It only worsened every symptom. The tens unit was unbearable, I sobbed while using it. The anti-inflammatories were of no help either.

I tried everything from nerve pain medications (Lyrica, Neurontin) to other anti-inflammatories designed for rheumatoid arthritis. My edema was so severe that my skin would be so tight that it would nearly weep. I began seeing another orthopedist and I asked for an amputation. I was desperate for relief.

Of course, this would simply add PLP to the dynamic. I requested joint replacements. I was told my bone density was so low due to the RSD damage that my bones would shatter with implants. (The surgeon had witnessed this before).

I had further testing, which revealed a lumbar lordosis and systemic bacterial infections caused by the RSD. I was exhausting my savings and credit cards. My insurance wasn't approving most. At this point, I had relocated, spent my savings on sliding shower chairs, wheelchair ramps, disability equipment (for eating, bathing, dressing, transferring, telephone, typing, etc.) travels to physicians, testing, etc., not covered by insurance due to the RSD.

Two years had now passed since my first symptom. I was drained emotionally, mentally, physically and financially. My boyfriend was now a nurse, not a significant other. He cooked, bathed me, dressed me, lifted me, trimmed my nails, and put my long hair in ponytails every day. Our romantic relationship had ended. We had transitioned to "patient and caregiver " as he poignantly stated. My spirit was crushed. He was exhausted. The little apartment we had been living in, which was to be temporary while I "healed from surgery and regained my life", was inappropriate for the long term. It was certainly not ADA. I decided to purchase a home in construction that we could modify to my needs. I wanted access to my bathroom, kitchen and outdoors! He did and so we moved again.... The second time in a year.

Another year of appointments, medicine trials, and testing would follow. I even ordered strange contraptions off the internet designed to help me walk on my own. I couldn't use them because my legs couldn't tolerate the straps. I resigned myself to a life of no ambulation, limited arm use (both shoulders were "frozen in place ") still with no hope as I was no longer a physical therapy candidate due to my poor bone density and the RSD. My new "normal" was an RSD patient who could not walk, had limited arm and hand use, could not chew solid food and exhausted easily after the conversation or movement.

I adapted quite well over the next decade. Yes, I had my moments!!! I went through every stage...denial, anger, resentment, etc.

Finally, I reached acceptance. More difficult than the RSD was knowing I was losing every aspect of my life as I knew it.

During the last decade, I slowly adapted my home: wheelchair ramps, specialty sinks with touch faucets, lower light switches, higher electrical outlets, lever door handles, lower thermostat with a smart app for my cell, remote control mini blinds, call bells for caregivers, adjustable Medical beds, etc. The list went on and on. This was my new normal. The specialists were of no more use and quite frankly that was fine with me as I was exhausted from traveling.

They each suggested that my PCP, who was local, could manage my symptoms as we all knew there was no cure and I had exhausted everything.

During the last 13-years, I tried physical therapy (traditional and aquatic), tens units, surgeries, nerve blocks, counseling, mirror therapy, medications (from anti-depressants to nerve pain inhibitors to anti-inflammatories) all for the prescribed duration. I had scheduled a ketamine infusion and reluctantly checked into the hospital in a small neighboring town, but didn't have peace about it and weighed all benefits and risks and decided it was simply too risky. I considered amputations, and joint replacements. I screamed, cried, prayed. I have to be honest, yes, I considered suicide.

In this time frame, my longtime boyfriend simply could no longer tolerate the life of a "nurse." Our romantic relationship had long been over and we had become roommates. We were both very unhappy. He couldn't take the stress any longer. I was devastated and terrified. Yet another thing this disease had taken from me. I was now forced to hire caregivers... Strangers...To be in my home during my most intimate of human moments. I was blessed to have a program that allowed me to hire my own employees. However, I was still devastated. If a person was a no show or called in sick, that meant I didn't eat that day or have hygiene.

THE BEAST HAD NOW TAKEN MY HEALTH, MY LEGS, MY INDEPENDENCE, MY CAREER, MY ABILITY TO EAT, SLEEPING, BATHING, FRIENDSHIPS, AND MY RELATIONSHIP. I WAS ALONE AND DISABLED.

Over the years, entrusting my body and home to strangers took its own toll. Having strangers, sometimes as many as four in a week, in my home was exhausting me in every aspect. I had ones that were so insensitive and insulted me. There were the ones who stole small items and I didn't bother reporting it as I needed the help. I have been sexually molested in my own bedroom. The epitome of criminal conduct was when a new hire stole all of my cherished jewelry (some of which once belonged to my Great Grandmother and Great Grandfather), my medications and my savings while threatening and extorting me. She had claimed to be an LPN for a local agency. She was employed by them. She had a clean background. I discovered she had no education and was not an LPN. However, she had spent her criminal career seeking her perfect victims.... Stroke patients or quadriplegics.

She sought outpatients who would not be aware or could not communicate her actions. I had her arrested the day I caught her stealing. I learned she had been doing so since her first week with me. This, of course, led to multiple statements by law officials in my bedroom. My nightmare of PTSD began. This was simply another physical issue to add to the RSD. I no longer trusted anyone. It in itself exacerbated my RSD to new extremes.

I accepted everything to the best of my ability. I found three pairs of pajama pants my legs would tolerate... On a good day. My wardrobe was now limited to eight items in total. I could not drive my car or leave my house unaided. I could not prepare food. I adapted to a nice life of being homebound with yogurt and baby food as staples. In the last decade, I saw my PCP usually two to five times a year and we found a handful of maintenance medications that allowed me some sleep, pain relief for bathing/hygiene and general comfort. This was by trial and error over 13-years. I lived my new normal until 2016.

In 2016, I began having intermittent episodes of debilitating vertigo. I had been complaining of episodes of dizziness for years with no solid answers from my PCP, ENT or Neurologist. The vertigo became more and more frequent and with it came severe anxiety as I literally could not keep my balance to sit or transfer. I literally could not sit up unaided to feed myself. For a year, I tried every medication for vertigo known to science. After a year, it rendered me bed-bound. My best guess is that somehow the blood flow restriction from the RSD had found its way into the vestibular system. This seemed perfectly plausible as it was obvious it had long since spread into my face and oral areas. I now had another horrific normal—bed-bound with 24-hour assistance required simply for basic ADLs (nutrition, toileting, and bathing).

Survival

A new issue now arose: how will I travel to my physician (a mere six miles away). If I even tried to transfer from my bed past my portable toilet, I became severely tachycardic and my oxygen level dropped. Over the past two years, it only intensified. I could no longer sit up in my car to travel, so I began seeking non-emergency ambulance transportation. This is very costly as insurance won't cover it. The least expensive I could find was a $470 round trip to my PCP six miles away. There was no choice, however, it was not successful. It took us 45-minutes to get me transferred and padded for the ride and we never made it past the entrance of my subdivision. At the entrance, I was severely tachycardic 160 bpm with a low 02 saturation and in severe pain from the vibration of the ambulance. Even though both paramedics called my PCP and explained traveling was unsafe, my PCP was unsympathetic and demanded an office visit. I attempted it again with my vehicle and two caregivers, I did get to the office. My pulse was 192 bpm on arrival. I thought I would have a stroke and die that day. This was the last time I was ever able to travel. This was in August of 2017.

THE ADVOCACY: "Shannon's Hope for House Calls & Home Medical Care" was born that day in Statesboro, GA.

During the past two years, my focus shifted to desperately searching for avenues to either travel to my physician or literally begging for him to make a house call. I was in the need for routine care and maintenance medications. I was told the House Calls were not permitted in Georgia. I naively believed my physician. My research showed otherwise.

I finally located a local ambulance transport who was equipped to meet my needs and agreed to transport if I signed a release as they felt it was unsafe and against my well-being to travel. They did, however, offer full paramedics and oxygen. The quote was $1,774.00 round trip (six miles one way). My friends started a fundraiser. Unfortunately, we never could raise the funds. My physician was kept abreast the entire time of all my attempts and avenues to see him for a visit.

I still attempted valiant efforts at transport. My health was declining and each attempt proved more detrimental to my health. It was now an intense struggle to transfer from my bed to a wheelchair without severe tachycardia, shortness of breath and a drastic drop in oxygen saturation. I left out a pivotal factor: My solar urticaria (allergy to the sunlight). I had battled it since I was 20-years old. It had now manifested in an allergy to artificial light. My immune system was now so weak that the antihistamines only dulled it to allow dim lighting, close to candlelight, even with medication. Caregivers, time and again, would say that we couldn't risk it and assisted me back to bed. They stated they couldn't be privy to such a detrimental attempt and refused to go further.

175

My last attempt was May of this year (2019). I had two caregivers and my Mother assisting. We had tried to plan for every detail. I valiantly made it from my bedroom to my foyer (via wheelchair).

My reaction was so intense that it was recorded on video. Again, tachycardic with a pulse of 165+ bpm, oxygen dropped (I had an oximeter in place) and the tremors were uncontrollable.

I was already developing hives from the daylight and natural light. My main caregiver wheeled me back and assisted me to the bed and laid me flat until I partially stabilized. Both caregivers were so distraught they asked to go to my appointment on my behalf and present the video...I gave consent. My physician watched the first 20-seconds & ignored the rest stating "I have seen 15,000 patients and I've never seen a patient who couldn't travel.

If she doesn't travel to me, she receives no more medications or care." This total lack of care or compassion was abhorrent.

He was privy to all of my efforts and showed only callous disregard. This was the last-straw.... Change had to occur, or I would lose my life!

I was now passionate to save my life and began reaching out to anyone who would listen in an attempt to advocate for House Calls.

A friend reached out via Facebook and offered to help knowing my limitations. She lives in Chicago, Illinois. The distance meant nothing, as she has been my ally, supporter, and confidant. She spent immeasurable man hour's emailing, calling and faxing on my behalf. We were soon collaborating with the Director of the CCSP in my State, University Professors in the Schools of Nursing and Sociology as well as Atlanta Legal Aid. Social Workers and Case Managers were of no avail whatsoever. We left no stone unturned.

My half-sibling had lost his life on Mother's Day of this same year after valiantly traveling to his physician and three separate emergency rooms for help for a severe UTI. (He had lost both legs, a hip and was paralyzed from an MVA early in life). He was 37-years old when he lost his battle. Even after multiple attempts at seeking routine medical care, he lost his life. This fueled my passion.

To add insult to injury, the very physician who had finally diagnosed my RSD was in medical school with my PCP. Hence, my PCP was keenly aware of my diagnosis and limitations. To simply state that every other patient could travel and there was no reason why traveling was of such detriment to me, and so painful, was insulting. He did, however, refer me to a local Hospice for palliative care. I went through an arduous assessment only to be denied as my records of 16-years with my PCP were so incomplete and vague. Also, they required more recent records of which I had none as I could no longer travel. I was referred to a second hospice only to have the same occur. It was a vicious "catch 22." Eventually, I was referred to a Palliative Agency an hour away in Savannah, GA. I, again, underwent an assessment only to be told they did not participate with my insurance. All of the before mentioned was an effort to bring care to me in my home. I now was truly faced with no other avenue but to find a House Call physician immediately.

Grueling months of mentally exhausting emails and calls revved into a pitch of panic. I had been involved with the latter for two years, but now the intensity was fierce. My body was so exhausted. The stress and fatigue only exacerbated the RSD. I could not give up! A contact from my dear friend in Chicago told me of a House Call Physician with an excellent reputation. He was sadly two hours away. My caregiver immediately called and explained briefly the situation. The receptionist suggested I write a detailed email of my needs, hx, etc.

Again, I shared my life with a stranger, pleading. There was no email reply. Weeks passed. I called to be told it's simply too far away. Desperation truly sets in. I was dividing my remaining medications now into 1/4 and 1/5 of the recommended dosage to stretch them as far as I possibly could. I could feel my body declining. I now decided to move to the final phase... I would pre-plan my final arrangements.

I cried, begged and pleaded to God for answers, help, and avenues to open. One morning, I was so weak, however, I felt led to look at Facebook at dawn (I had not slept from pain and worry). The very first post on my Newsfeed was from the House Call Physician's page (I had "liked" them months ago to have another avenue of communication). They were "LIVE!" I saw that little green light, and commented immediately. It was a very sincere comment stating I so wished they served my area as I desperately needed care.

The PA replied to me personally!! He commented to call that afternoon and I did. This was my Miracle. He returned my call that afternoon at 6:00 p.m. and spoke with my caregiver for 30-minutes.

He was gracious, polite and caring. He stated he was not very familiar with RSD, but he would research and call me back the next day (which was Saturday). He did...promptly at 6:00 pm! This led to a third call on Monday during which he/we coordinated a home visit appointment. Insurance would pay for the appointment. The travel time would be out of pocket. He would need to set aside five-hours for me (four-hours of travel round trip and an hour visit). I was elated. I used the funds my friends had raised earlier for the attempted non-ambulance transport. This was God. A miracle!

The day I had been praying and hoping for arrived. I had a House Call! He arrived with his nurse. They were kind, caring and professional. They were understanding of my extreme sensitivity to touch and sounds. All of my limitations from RSD were respected. This in itself was monumental. I had my exam, to the extent my body allowed. I even had an EKG. Due to the extreme nature and cost, this could only occur rarely. However, I was on my way to another "new normal..." One that would literally save my life!

It was now time to breathe and focus on my health and initiating this as a permanent means of medical care for myself and all others in my area. Months earlier I had started following a page on Facebook for mobile phlebotomy (blood draws). They were too far away to service my area. I "liked" every page I could find on Facebook regarding mobile medical care as you never know where help will originate. Within weeks of my house call, I received a message from the mobile phlebotomy company asking if I was still in need of service. I responded instantly... YES!! I then began coordinating with the owner, via Facebook, to coordinate with her and find a local lab who would coordinate with us all. As I type this sentence, I'm literally awaiting an appointment for home serology.

I never would have imagined 13-years ago, when I first became unable to bear weight and walk, this would be my life. I'm thankful I didn't know my future as I honestly don't think my heart and mind could have borne the burden. At my first introduction to RSD, even before my official diagnosis, I was devastated. I could not stop sobbing. I had never faced anything where there was no "fix." This beast had no cure and progressed. I thought to myself "if I can no longer bear this, I can always end my life." This actually brought me peace as it gave me a mental option where there was none in reality. God was merciful and this "hell", as I call it, was gradual. This allowed me to keep my sanity as I never knew the next step would be more intense and more quality of life would be lost. The not knowing was my saving grace.

Today, I feel my purpose is to create a legacy and hope from my heartbreak, pain, and losses. I lost every dream and aspect of a normal life to RSD. Survival was my goal for the past 13-years. My dreams of being a Veterinarian were dashed.

After I completed my BBA in Accounting (focus in forensic as my Alma Mater is the only accredited University in the Country to offer this subfield hence my further feeling of accomplishment), my career as a Forensic Accountant was dashed. God had other plans. I am now here to initiate hope for all others living with the same struggles. May I pave a new road of home-delivered medical care to my area is my aspiration and prayer.

This is the story of how "Shannon's Hope for House Calls & Home Care" was born. I hope to have the strength to manage a website and Facebook page. I'm currently reaching out to local physicians hoping to recruit someone who is willing and has the heart to care for the zebras of the world even if the Hoofbeats sound like horses!

NEVER GIVE UP! NEVER!

My story is one of survival. The literal fight to survive. Survival when the only person in this fight was me. May we all have a future of hope from the struggles!

Best wishes to all and God bless you!!

~Shannon

MY CRPS JOURNEY
By: Elizabeth VanScoter

June of 2010 was like any other summer day. Until I had an accident that caused a tiny fracture of my tibia. I went to an orthopedic doctor, and he put on a pretty purple cast. When that cast came off six weeks later, oddly, my leg looked worse than when the cast was put on. While the bruising had resolved, my leg was more swollen and red. My doctor was concerned about a blood clot, so he sent me for an ultrasound. What was found started me down a path I never expected.

The ultrasound tech completed the test, taking all sorts of measurements and such. Afterward, she took me back to the waiting room and told me my doctor was going to call me. My doctor called me immediately and said a large blood clot was found in my thigh. I had to start on shots given in my belly immediately.

When I went back to my doctor a few days later for a recheck, he repeatedly said he did not like how my leg looked. He also wanted me to start physical therapy (PT). At my first appointment, the PT said they had never seen so much swelling. My PT also said he suspects he knows what I have, but he didn't want to tell me out of fear I would research it.

My doctor sent me to pain management in December of 2010 and that's the first time I heard the term complex regional pain syndrome (CRPS) - and what I didn't know was how much that diagnosis would permanently alter my life.

That started me on a path of nerve blocks, bier blocks, serial casting, physical therapy, too many medications to recall, tests, surgeries, wound care, many different specialty doctors, including the Cleveland Clinic and a world-renowned doctor in Philadelphia. I felt like a guinea pig because each doctor I saw said my case was one of the most severe they have ever seen. Most gave me the feeling I already had – helpless.

I had a spinal cord stimulator (SCS) and intrathecal pain pump put in. While both initially were somewhat helpful, my CRPS raged on and wiped out any treatment in its path.

I was willing to try anything because the constant excruciating pain was (is) unbearable. Nothing was providing any significant relief; meanwhile, the swelling was getting worse. The swelling had become so bad that my leg was no longer able to contain all the fluids, and I started getting fracture blisters/open sores. As the swelling worsens, so do the skin ulcers. Since the skin on my leg is never able to heal, I started having recurring bouts of cellulitis that landed me in the hospital for a week or more each time with several I.V. Antibiotics constantly running. After a year of that, my primary doctor started discussing amputation because he said it is just a matter of time before the next infection will not respond and it will be fatal. I was not ready to give in, though. I battled for another year, with many more hospitalizations for cellulitis. I knew my leg would never recover any function by this point – it was totally deformed, grossly swollen, with huge open and infected areas. After a lot of vacillating I let them amputate my left leg (below the knee) on May 31, 2017.

While I suffer silently, my family bears the real burden. My three girls have had to miss out on events, see things they shouldn't have to see and grow up faster than they were supposed to. My husband has had to pick up the slack for things I can no longer do. I should be able to go help my mother, and it breaks my heart that I cannot.

I've been left a former shell of what I once was. I've become a master at disguising the constant excruciating pain. But I'm still here, so I suppose that's considered a win….

KATE HIBBERT'S CRPS STORY
By: Kate Hibbert

Trying to condense 19-years of medical history and life into a short piece of writing is not easy! Some defining moments can't be listed as a dot point, but I'll try to share what I can, what I take out of the 19-years.

I was diagnosed with complex regional pain syndrome (CRPS) in late 2000, after a botched blood test on my right arm (inner elbow). I knew straight away that it didn't feel "right," I looked down and saw the needle was almost at a 90° angle to my arm. The "nurse" had put the needle through the vein and into my median nerve, causing the most immense pain. I screamed at her to take the needle out, but she shushed me and told me it would be over in a second. Normally, your nerves aren't the source of your pain, they merely send the pain signals from one part of your body to your brain. For the nerves themselves to be injured is like having a giant, open-cut along your arm, then putting a burning hot poker in the middle of that cut and wriggling it around... A lot. That's CRPS in a nutshell.

And so, it began. At the time I was a new wife and mum, living in Newcastle, Australia, with my husband and our two young daughters, aged 2.5-years old and seven months old. Parenting babies and toddlers, one-armed was near impossible. I had been back and forth to my doctor about how much pain I was in, with them saying to come back in a few weeks if it didn't get better, which it didn't, so after a few months I was able to see a pain specialist (something I had never heard of until then). He said Yep, you have CRPS (well, it was more commonly known as reflex sympathetic dystrophy (RSD) back then). There's no effective treatment and no cure. Sadly, you can expect to be in a wheelchair within one year. Here are some opioids, off you go.

Hearing that was devastating, I was 23-years old, I didn't want that to be my future! I searched the internet for more information but because it was 2001, the internet was a baby, especially in terms of medical information. There were very few sites that discussed CRPS and how to treat it. Doctor Hooshmand's "RSD Puzzles" were the only source of useful information in terms of treatment options and understanding the condition. I first got in contact with Eric Phillips and Doctor Hooshmand back in 2001, when I found out that the way my CRPS started, from a Venipuncture (blood test or IV needle) injury, is not at all common... Lucky me!

Finding doctors and medical practitioners that not only knew about CRPS but also knew the "do's and don'ts" of rehabilitating a CRPS limb and keeping it strong was a constant struggle for me, especially as we moved a lot over the years. Many said CRPS is all psychological, some said I didn't have CRPS because, especially in the early days, I had no visible symptoms. My hand and arm would swell at times, but of course never when I was in a doctor's office! It's frustrating when you wait for months to see a doctor that supposedly knows CRPS and the treatment options, then you finally see them and they offer no help. But there are more and more doctors and physios now that DO know how to treat CRPS so the important thing to do is to keep going until you find one.

In the first few months of my diagnosis, when most of the internet information said that CRPS is a downhill slope to total disability within a year, I did manage to find a chat room devoted to CRPS called Braintalk and it was amazing to talk to others who were in the same situation as me with this monster. They hadn't all deteriorated in the manner I had read about, some had had CRPS for years and were still able to walk around and function every day. That gave me hope! I'm still very close friends with the people I met on that forum, 19-years later. The support they gave me when no one else in my "real" world knew what CRPS was or what it's like to be diagnosed with an incurable condition. That connection to other CRPS'ers got me through each day. Over the years, my online support network expanded to a whole range of forums and websites all over the world. I became involved in an Australian group in 2002 that helped me through so many of my dark days and got excited as my family grew. There is nothing better than connecting with other CRPS'ers- whether they're in your neighborhood or across the world. You feel less isolated and more understood- two feelings that are intrinsic in not letting CRPS beat you.

My husband and I didn't want my CRPS to define our life and our future, so before my condition deteriorated any further, we decided to have "one more baby", as we had always wanted three or four kids. Some called us crazy, but we felt it was worth the risk. Luckily for me, that was a great decision! In late 2001, I fell pregnant with my son and amazingly, my CRPS went into total remission during the whole pregnancy- no pain, no medications needed- it all just vanished! So, I threw myself into Physio and strengthening exercises and playing with my daughters while I could. It was an amazing break! But within hours of his birth, my pain came back, bigger and worse than ever. I couldn't breastfeed him, I couldn't even have his blanket touch my right arm, so I had to go back on my medications. But then my body threw me another curve ball. I had a dangerous allergic reaction to the medication that had helped me so much before my pregnancy. It was scary. It didn't make sense. It was devastating. Now I had three kids under the age of four, I was one-armed again and having to start trying new meds at the same time. But I wasn't giving in. I learned to write left-handed, I learned to change a nappy on a toddler one-armed and to do the buttons up on jeans one-handed!

My husband had to quit his full-time job in 2002 and become the full-time career for myself and the kids. It wasn't easy, but I was grateful for his help and he loved being home with us, watching the kids grow up. When my pain was being fairly well managed, I threw myself into Physio again- clenching my fist four times one day, then five times the next day and so on. That's the only way to do it. Push yourself but not to the brink. That's one thing I learned with all the hours of Physio and treatments and pain management classes and knowing my body- push yourself but stop at 80%, not 100% or 120%- you just can't do that with CRPS. Maybe start at 60% of what you think you can do, then build up from there. Going all out at 120% just causes more harm than good! The recovery time, the higher pain levels... You don't gain anything from that. I used that mentality many times in the past 19-years.

In 2004, I had my first seven-day inpatient ketamine infusion. These were the early days of ketamine infusions. At that point, very few places in the US were trialing them, but I found a specialist in Australia who was trialing them and I begged to be included. The pain relief was almost immediate, my kids (who were now ages 6, 4, and 2) could touch my right arm and hand for the first time ever. That was a HUGE moment! The first time I had had any hope in a long time. The total pain and symptom relief lasted 30 amazing days, then when it wore off, I went back into hospital for another infusion. That one broke a record! I was the first person in Australia to get more than six months of total remission from a ketamine infusion! As we neared the seven months, my husband and I decided to have that "One More baby" (yeah, I know, we don't learn!) We figured that even if the pain came back, I could have another infusion after the baby was born and I'd be fine. Unfortunately, it didn't go that way.

One of the joys of being in Australia is the lovely spiders you share your house with. When I was seven months pregnant with my daughter Hannah, still benefiting from the infusion, I was bitten on my right leg by a white tail spider. The pain and nerve damage that came from that bite on my leg seemed to "wake up" my arm from its hibernation. I was then left with full-blown CRPS in my right arm- shoulder to fingertips-and my right leg- toes to the thigh, with no medications I could take that was safe for pregnancy. I became reliant on crutches to go from one room to the next, my kids had to carry things for me and help me get around. It was a soul-destroying time for me, I have to admit. A relapse and a spread weren't part of our plan.

When my daughter was about eight weeks old, I went into the hospital for my third ketamine infusion, the one we pinned all our hopes on. Unfortunately, that time it didn't work, not only did I not receive any pain relief or signs of remission, my liver stopped functioning properly so the infusion was stopped after the third day. I was devastated. I couldn't walk without crutches but I couldn't hold the crutch with my right hand- I was stuck. Now I had a newborn baby as well as three kids. Thankfully, we had an amazing support network around us and my husband and I just did what we had to do and found ways to enjoy the simple moments when we could.

So, I got back on the merry-go-round of trying different drug combinations to find a treatment plan that helped. Over the years, I found that a combination of opioids, antidepressants and muscle relaxants helped the most. Sometimes one would be on a higher dose and other times another was. I'd swap from MS Contin to Oxycodone every six to twelve months, as I found they both took the higher pain levels away, but had different side effects on the rest of my body, so a rotation worked well. I never wanted to take more than I needed so I would reassess every few months. But I found a way to get by, so I could walk around the house and shower without help.

I went on to have more ketamine infusions and got great relief from them, some let me lower my pain meds by half for four to six months, which gave my body a much-needed break from high levels of drugs, but I was chasing a result I never achieved again. I had my eleventh ketamine infusion two years ago- the short-lasting pain relief wasn't worth the cost of being away from my family for a week.

But I didn't give up. I studied from home when my pain was lessened. I completed two tertiary qualifications from home, over seven years. It wasn't easy, but I never gave up hope that one day I would be able to work again. That's what I worked towards-always believing that another new treatment option is just around the corner so prepare yourself for that day!

But nothing ever goes smoothly with CRPS, that's the only predictable part of it! I sprained my "bad" ankle in 2009 and that caused a massive flare up and swelling issue that took months to crawl back from. But I did.

I bent my "bad" wrist awkwardly in 2011, and broke it, which caused a huge flare-up and massive swelling. I was so medicated I don't remember much of the four months that followed, but I remember the crying and how twisted my hand was. I thought "That's it, I had a good run, I fought a good fight, the best is behind me, this is my reality and I have to accept it." But I kept fighting anyway!

To get me through, I once again learned to write left-handed. I used crossword puzzles to help me keep the lettering, small and even. I worked hard to untwist my hand and I gained a lot of function back. Things were looking up.

But then, in 2010, my world turned upside down. My three eldest kids were in a horrific freeway crash. My second daughter, Olivia, didn't survive. All of a sudden, my CRPS wasn't the worst thing to happen to me anymore. I had to focus on my family and just do whatever I needed to do to be able to function and look after my kids each day. I raised my meds to a point where they helped a great deal without any bad side effects. My family needed me to be able to not just function day to day, but to be able to hug them, carry them, lie awkwardly in a single bed for hours with them while they struggled to fall asleep and stay asleep. I had to fight against the CRPS to have control over my body so that I could be the mum my kids needed me to be, whilst also working through my grief and PTSD. As I said, it turned our lives upside down, but we clung on to each other and had an amazing amount of support from my family, our friends, and my CRPS family around the world. That support kept me going.

In 2012, I was on a steady treatment plan that let me do light housework here and there, but I only had a couple of functioning hours each day. I couldn't get groceries, I couldn't vacuum, I couldn't drive them to their medical appointments or school. I needed crutches when I left the house. I decided I wanted to do more. I was sick of slowing down my kids or having to watch from the sidelines, so I started walking. You've probably heard of the "Couch to 5km" programs, to get couch potatoes off their butts and onto a treadmill? Mine was a literal couch to 5k program. My lounge room was 5m long, so four times a day, I walked from one wall to the next, trying to keep my feet even and not limp. I then extended it to four times a day, walking back and forth four times. Once I was doing better at that, I bought a second-hand treadmill. I was scared of walking down the street in case I went too far and couldn't walk back again, so the treadmill was the perfect option. I wanted to do more, but the pain was getting too much so my doctor agreed to raise one of my medications for six months so I could exercise and build up my strength, then lower my meds down after that time.

I slowly built up my strength and mobility and after nine months (three months after lowering my meds back down again), I walked/jogged a 5km fun run with my eldest daughter! She had never seen me so well.

Apart from the remissions during my 2002 pregnancy and the benefit of my second ketamine infusion in 2005, I had always been disabled to her. To jog over the finish line, hand in hand, when I'd been so limited for so long, was huge. It was 12-years into my RSD, I wasn't meant to be able to run!

Since then, my lack of motor skills and coordination have caused me to have more broken bones, sprained joints, and crazy flare-ups. My CRPS spread to my left arm after an I.V. site for my ninth ketamine infusion caused an infection, which caused nerve damage in my hand. That was hard to cope with- adjusting to having both arms, and my leg affected.

In 2016, after a long period of putting my health on the back burner- just giving it the attention it needed to keep going, but nothing more than that- I decided to start an exercise plan again, but I was still recovering from sprain and strain injuries so I couldn't walk without crutches, so this time I started in a heated hydrotherapy pool. I'd do the same as I had done in my lounge years before- go from one wall to the other. The first week or so, I was barely in the pool for ten minutes each time, but it was where I had to start. Gradually I could walk a couple of laps across the pool (10m). Then I started using weights and floaties to build my muscles up. Bit by bit is the only way to fight CRPS.

I wrote everything down each day so I could slowly see my progression. Again, I didn't push myself past my limit, but I stopped before I got to it, which is hard to do when you just want to move! But it was the only way for me so that I wasn't on a constant roller coaster of too much exercise causing massive flare-ups then over-exercising again after the pain lessened. I found I didn't gain anything by pushing myself like that. It's an endgame thing. Anyway, my work in the pool got me back to being able to walk on a treadmill, which got to the point where I could run, and I mean RUN, 7kms every day!

I'm not saying this to be arrogant or cocky, I just want to motivate others to not give up, to make those little steps and to work for the end game. I've had loads of downtimes, where I'm back to being on crutches full time or unable to put my arms up and wash my hair, but I didn't give in.

In 2017, my left leg joined the party. There was no trigger for that spread though, no injury, I just started having symptoms in that leg. I now have full-body CRPS, with all of my organs and nervous systems affected too. It's been a mental battle that I haven't always won. CRPS is a third person in your marriage, it's the conjoined twin that, more often than not, gets the final say in what you can do and how you feel. It is so much easier to give in to you CRPS than to fight it. It's exhausting to take two steps forward when CRPS keeps pushing you three steps back, but you have to keep trying. If I didn't keep trying all those times, I wouldn't have my two post-CRPS babies, I wouldn't have had the eight-month ketamine remission, I wouldn't have experienced doing 7km runs every day through beautiful bushland. And I wouldn't have had the fun moments with my kids while they were young.

What helped me with my mental health was starting up a local CRPS support group with a friend. We had both been to a local one run by a pain clinic that was finishing up, and it was suggested we start our community support group so that anyone can come, not just patients of the private pain clinic. We did just that, we put out advertisements in local doctors' clinics, in hospital waiting rooms, all over our region's Facebook pages, and we were shocked at how many people responded. In our town, we have more than 80 CRPS'ers! So much for it being a rare condition!

We started meeting twice a month-either going out for coffee or lunch or having guest speakers talk to us. I wanted to bring specialists to our members that they may not be able to access themselves due to financial or transportation reasons. So, we had myotherapists, Hypnotherapists, art therapists, physios, laser light therapists, pain specialists, Pilates instructors, dieticians, nutritionists... Every specialist that felt that they could help us was welcome, and they all donated their time and skills! It's been three years since CRPSgeelong began and the friendships that have come from that group have been life-changing for all of our members. So many isolated suffers who felt that no one understood them found that they weren't alone. Knowing I had a hand in that is amazing.

One goal that has remained with me since I was diagnosed was to have a job again, to have a career, to contribute to the world and to my family, after my husband had so much pressure on him for so long to work full time and look after the kids and me. A year ago, I had a spinal cord stimulator trial. I'd put it off for many years as my history with needles and cuts wasn't a good one, but I was confident in the new technology and wanted to give it a go. Apart from the expected surgical pain, the stimulator worked well. I'm hoping to get the permanent stim put in at some point, but the timing isn't right at the moment. When I had that trial done, I couldn't wear pants. I couldn't have any fabric touch my right leg or foot, it was a nightmare, but other than that, my pain wasn't too bad. I decided I wanted to see if there was any work I could do. Even when my leg was bad, I could sit in front of a laptop and type quickly. My brain and my fingers worked well enough to do that. I decided I'd go into my husband's office a couple of times a week to help with general office tasks, for an hour or two at a time. I loved it! I slowly built up my stamina, juggled my pain meds and spent a lot of time doing Physio for my right leg, with the touch sensitivity. I injured my right ankle badly in early 2019, tearing ligaments on both sides, and in front, my right ankle. The flare-up from that was excruciating and the recovery was slow, it's still slow. But I kept going. I went to temping jobs on crutches, with a moon boot on, after all, once I was sitting down, I was no different to anyone else! Those short jobs were amazing to do, no matter how mundane they were. So, where did my stubbornness get me?

To now, 19-years since my CRPS began, I am working full time for the first time! I work in a busy university, as a business support officer, doing admin, accounts, fleet management, data entry, contractor inductions, field trip organizations and more. I love it! They know about my CRPS but it hasn't been a problem so far. I get to sit on a soft and comfortable seat, in a well-heated (but not too heated!) office. My car parking spot, my office, and the canteen are all within about 15-meters, so my lack of mobility isn't a problem.

They're accommodating on my bad days, but I'm mostly able to manage to get through the day. The muscle fatigue builds up, so I'm shattered by the end of the day but it's worth it. I don't know how long I'll last like this, CRPS is so unpredictable, but I'll ride this wave as long as it lasts! Not only are my crutches not in my car anymore, but they're also not even in the house- they're in my garage! I still manage my pain, it's full body now, so the full-body muscle aches and fatigue are my biggest challenge, but I just have to pace myself. I'm doing more than I ever thought I could be doing this far into my CRPS.

There's so much more I can say, so many milestones in my CRPS journey, good and bad, but what I'm wanting to get across is that CRPS isn't always a downhill slide to full-body CRPS where you're totally dependent on others and in extreme pain. It can be a roller coaster too. I've had the low lows where I thought I was past my best days, but then you find yourself thinking "Wait, I couldn't do this movement/activity a few months ago" and you smile a little and enjoy the moment. That then spurs you on to make that moment last as long as possible and create more!

I don't know for sure that a cure for CRPS will ever be found, but I'm planning and preparing for that day anyway. The amount of knowledge that scientists, researchers, and doctors (the good ones!) have about CRPS now compared to when I was diagnosed in 2000, is unbelievable. There was no talk of glia cells or central sensitization back then! The information was extremely limited, but it's not now and I'm very thankful for that! I know that some really good treatment options that everyone can access and benefit from are just around the corner. I know that scientists around the world have spent years studying this condition and I'm so grateful for that. That spurs me on and I hope it spurs you on, too. Don't think that a CRPS diagnosis means the end of your life as you know it- it just means you'll have to work hard, taking one tiny step after the next, until you can take bigger ones and until more effective treatment options become available to us.

My kids are now aged 21, 17, and 13 and I'm a Nana to a precious little girl. Life has been hard, but it's been worth it. Raising four kids with my husband- having two post-CRPS pregnancies and babies- and running the support group have been big achievements for sure, but my biggest achievement is being able to wear pants again when I couldn't this time last year. Anyone with CRPS knows that's something you don't take for granted!

ONE OF THE BEST AND WORST DAYS OF MY LIFE
By: Brenna Fletcher

My story is a little long and I believe it is all-important to understand the extent of my frustration, pain, and suffering so please bear with me. Thank you in advance for your time.

On May 03, 2019, I was diagnosed with complex regional pain syndrome (CRPS) due to an improperly administered spinal anesthesia. This is the day I knew my life would never be the same. That I would live every day here on out with unrelenting pain.

On May 18, 2018, I had a repeat c-section to deliver my son. Six years earlier, I was forced to have an emergency c-section at the same hospital to deliver my daughter. An emergency c-section was required the first time because they waited until I was past my due date to do an ultrasound to check her, even though I had been telling them for a week before her due date that she was breech and I could feel her head in my ribs. When they finally did check it was already too late. She was breech, had very little fluid and had to be delivered ASAP. She was delivered that afternoon and I later came to find out she is autistic.

Therefore, due to the previous birth, this was a repeat c-section and was scheduled. When they were prepping me, a female anesthesiologist came in to talk to me about the procedure. I informed her that she may have a tough time with my anesthesia because the first time (six years earlier) they had a hard time finding where exactly to put the needle. They ended up having to have their best anesthesiologist do it, but ultimately, they did find the right spot and I had no complications. She made a joke about she thought her kids needed her and she may have to leave (because she really did not want to do it), she then laughed and was like well if I can't get it then there is another anesthesiologist here who has been here a long time and he SHOULD be able to do it.

When it came time for the anesthesia, they inserted the needle and began trying to find the spot. Extreme pain started shooting down either one leg or the other as they dug the needle around. I was asked to tell them which side I was feeling the pain in as I was crying my eyes out because it hurt so bad. (I have since read that there should be no pain and that if the patient feels pain, they are supposed to stop immediately.) I would tell them one side they would move the needle then it would be the other side. This continued for a while (23-minutes to be exact), with them digging the needle around in my back as I cried and told them which leg, they were causing pain to shoot down. I am not sure how many times they tried or how many people tried as I was instructed to hug a nurse in front of me and was sitting on the edge of a table in intense pain and unable to stop crying. Eventually, they said okay, you are going to feel a zing. I was still telling them that I was feeling the pain down my left leg, but I don't know if they were tired of searching or just thought it was "close enough" because they said oh it should be okay and the "zing" was coming. At this point, they injected the anesthesia and it was definitely a ZING. I screamed in pain as my left leg kicked straight out, off the table, on its own and was instantly filled with the worst pain I had ever felt in my life. Shortly after the anesthesia kicked in and I was numb.

So, it was time to begin the c-section. My husband and a nurse were beside my head, and I began telling them I could not breathe. I remember clearly that I honestly thought I was going to die. I struggled to tell them I couldn't breathe over and over. It is kind of a blur at this point the nurse was telling me it was a normal side effect of the anesthesia (which the first time I had had one I was cold and got the shakes, this was completely different) I felt as though she was not taking me seriously.

My husband said she asked if I wanted air and gave me some through the hoses that go in your nose. All I remember is struggling to repeatedly tell them I couldn't catch my breath. Even when they pulled my son out and held him up for me to see and then tried to lay him against me, I couldn't enjoy it or take in the moment. I thought I was going to die. (I know I said that a few times, but it was the scariest thing I had ever experienced. Until the following week.) I now believe with the improperly placed spinal the anesthesia had traveled up my spine as well, causing the breathing problems that were brushed off by the nurse. Problems that could have killed me.

As the anesthesia wore off, I slowly began to be able to breathe again and the intense pain returned to my left leg. The pain was awful in my leg, the pain from being cut open was nowhere near the pain in my leg. It was extremely swollen and looked bruised. They did scans to make sure I did not have a blood clot and then a male anesthesiologist came and spoke to me. He said that they did have a hard time positioning the needle and "well, we might have scratched or irritated some nerves" he acted like no big deal you should feel better in a couple of weeks. I was released to go home after the normal amount of time, still in pain and unsure of why.

When my son was six days old, he developed a high fever and we rushed him to the ER. There I had to watch my barely a week-old baby had to undergo a spinal tap to check him for meningitis. I had to stand there and help hold down my naked screaming newborn as he went through having a big needle poked in his tiny back in the same place that just put me in all this pain a week earlier. It was heartbreaking. It came back that he did have viral meningitis that he contracted at the hospital the day he was born (it takes six to seven days for viral meningitis symptoms to present). Viral meningitis is not treatable and we were told it was between him and God whether he would make it or not. He was hooked up to I.V.'s and heart monitors for days. It was awful, we prayed and prayed. He was a little fighter and after a few days he was improving. We were again released from the hospital.

Back home it had now been two weeks and the pain in my left leg was no better. It is a constant burning, sometimes shooting like lightning strikes, pain.

The top of my foot is hypersensitive. The slightest breeze or bed sheet touching it sends pain shooting up my leg. The side of my big toe is completely numb, and the sole is also extra sensitive. I did not know who to call so I started with my OBGYN who told me if it was not C-Section cut related there was nothing they could do. They said I could try going back to the ER, maybe I could talk to the anesthesiologist? They didn't know. Well, it isn't like anesthesiologists have offices and after all, I had been through in the past two weeks, I certainly did not want to go back to the hospital a third time or have to leave my son. I believed it would just take a little longer to heal and I could tough it out, I thought surely it would get better that is what they had told me.

After a few months of it not getting any better, being in continuous pain with my leg, ankle and foot swelling daily, I went to see my primary care doctor I have seen for many years. He referred me to a neurologist. I went to see her multiple times, have had a total of three MRIs and an EMG. The second MRI noted degenerative changes in the area correlating to where the nerves are damaged at only eight months later.

Around April of 2019, the pain intensified. By night time I am in so much pain, I just curl up in my bed and cry. Some days are worse than others, if it is cold or rainy the pain is awful all day long. If I am up standing on it or trying to do things the pain shoots through my back, down my hip, leg, and calf and over the top of my foot. Walking on my foot when the pain intensifies feels like my foot is shattered. There are also spots where I feel like I am being stabbed. I sweat profusely. Sitting, standing or lying in certain positions for any period causes my foot to go numb and tingle. I have electrical shock feelings that course through my foot and leg. I feel as if I have something crawling on me at times when nothings there. The muscles, especially in my calf jerk and spasm when I lay down. My leg feels stiff and weak. Sometimes the pain, even appears in other parts of my body as well as both legs, my left shoulder, and neck along with my arms and hands. At times I am in so much pain that my blood pressure skyrockets, I cannot catch my breath, my lips and teeth feel tingly and numb, my ears ring and my head feels as if it's floating. I have a hard time concentrating, my memory is worse, I cannot stand temperature changes, if it is the least bit hot, I am drenched in sweat. My leg, ankle and foot swell and sometimes it looks black and blue, sometimes red and there is an indention in my calf. The skin on the top of my foot looks shiny, is often warmer or cooler than the opposing side and is still hypersensitive. The outside of my big toe is still numb. I still did not have a diagnosis or know what was wrong with me. At my last neurologist appointment (May 3, 2019) it was rainy and I was having a flare-up. I was limping, pouring sweat, my blood pressure was through the roof. I tried to hold back the tears of pain and frustration of all this time searching for an answer and some relief as I told her again how much pain I was in and how I didn't understand if it was just something that was rare or they did not want to admit what happened with my anesthesia or what. She told me that nobody was trying to deny what happened with my spinal anesthesia or what they had done, and it was all in my charts. She then went on to diagnose me with radicular dystrophy or RSD-CRPS at that appointment. She would not let me drive in the condition I was in and I was instructed to go to the ER. After an awful visit there when I did finally see a doctor, he told me it was too hard on my body to keep putting it through that much pain and I needed to be in pain management ASAP.

On June 18, 2019, I finally saw a pain management specialist and he also said it was CRPS Type II (causalgia) due to the spinal anesthesia. I am in severe pain every day over something I was told should feel better in a couple of weeks and could have been avoided had they just stopped when I was in that much pain and tried something different. I never was in labor they had plenty of time. Instead, it was brushed aside when had they paid attention, I may have been able to get the treatment that would have stopped it to progressing to what it is now, irreversible. My OBGYN office did not even call me to set up an appointment for a six week after my delivery checkup. I feel as though I was brushed off by everyone, especially the anesthesiologists who gave me a lifelong nerve condition when I went in to have a baby and have been suffering ever since.

I have a seven-year-old autistic daughter, and a year-old baby to take care of and not only has it put me in physical but also emotional pain. I can no longer do things that I used to love. I cannot be the mother or the wife, I used to be or I want to be because of the intense pain. I am even struggling to find a pain management clinic to even help me manage the pain as the first one I saw only wanted to put a spinal cord stimulator into my back, which I do not want. I am 30-years old and disabled.

I now have the most painful condition known to man that I will have the rest of my life and could lead to the loss of my leg, because they continually stuck a needle in my back even after I was in unimaginable pain, hoping to find the right spot over and over again. In doing so, they damaged those nerve roots and tissue, causing the CRPS. I had no idea this event was even a possible outcome of the spinal anesthesia. Why didn't they stop instead of not thinking twice about repeatedly poking a big needle into a very delicate spot in someone's back? They should have known what could happen, but in the end, they aren't the ones who will have to deal with this pain every single minute of every single day. My whole life has been forever changed because of what should have been one of the happiest days of my life.

OCCUPATIONAL THERAPIST NEEDS THERAPY
By: Kimberly Towles

March 19, 2009, started like any other day. I was a 39-year old occupational therapist working at a small outpatient clinic attached to a small hospital in a small town. I was happily married with two kids (my son was 16 and my daughter was 11). I was teaching my patient how to safely get in and out of his power wheelchair to get in and out of his van. He backed up onto my right foot and when I yelped, he changed directions and drove forward again. My foot began to hurt and immediately swelled inside my shoe. I could prop it up and put ice on it right away. After an hour or so, the pain was different. It just felt "off." I was sent to an orthopedic doctor who did X-rays and saw no fractures or dislocations, just swelling. I was put in a walking boot and sent back to work. I wore the boot for about three weeks and was able to wear my regular shoes again. By June I was having pain following the peroneal nerve path and put in a cast shoe and started physical therapy (PT). By July my foot started to show a purplish discoloration and I was having pain in the ball of my foot with walking. Occasionally the pain felt like I was stepping on a hot nail that was being driven through the ball of my foot. My doctor mentioned that my foot was showing some signs of complex regional pain syndrome (CRPS). I was started on Lyrica and began to wear a compression sock to help with pain and swelling. I had my first two sympathetic nerve blocks in June 2009. The color change was now up to mid-calf. I had a nerve conduction study in July that year that showed neuropathy of the peroneal nerve. At this time, I was started on Neurontin, and I was still working full time, using a knee scooter or wheelchair to control the pain.

By August I was having pain that was like wearing a barbed wire sock. My foot and ankle alternated from icy hot to raging fire with no reason for one or the other. I was removed from work for three weeks to let my pain come under control and get to my first appointment with pain management.

The doctor at pain management confirmed the diagnosis of CRPS. I was in shock that I was being diagnosed with what I had only heard about briefly in school; and, at the same time, relieved that what I was feeling had a true name and treatment plan. I had my first and second lumbar sympathetic nerve blocks in September. I was allowed to go back to work on a modified schedule of three days a week for a month after that. My third lumbar sympathetic block was in October and gave relief for about 24-hours. My foot was still swollen and changing from icy hot to raging fire for no apparent reason.

The stress was starting to affect me with crying spells at home and work. I was feeling like I was going in circles, letting everyone down. I was sent to work with a pain psychologist in November, eight months after my injury. I was diagnosed with reactive clinical depression.

In March 2010, I had my trial for a spinal cord stimulator (SCS) because I was continuing to have pain that was not controlled with medications or PT. Initially, I had fair relief with the stimulator and my pain would come and go. A CT scan was done that showed no problems in my lower back that would cause the pain I did have. By August I was having back spasms and pain had spread to my right knee and hip. The back spasms continued to get worse and I was having to arch my back to feel the stimulator work.

In September, I had my stimulator leads exchanged for a paddle and thoracic laminectomy. This surgery was complicated by scar tissue, causing the paddle to flex and bend, bruising my spinal cord and making me spend five days in the hospital on a cooling bed along with I.V. Steroids to stop swelling of my spinal cord. I had a systemic reaction to the adhesive used during the surgery that sent me back to the operating room to rule out infection. My life felt out of control. I was in my early forties and using a cane to get around. I wasn't able to work in my career that I loved and my social life consisted of pool exercise classes I was attending with retirees at the YMCA.

I was diagnosed with insomnia, anxiety, and panic attacks all related to CRPS. I began several months of passing blood in my urine and after having a cystoscopy and biopsy I was diagnosed with interstitial cystitis. My urologist referred to it as "CRPS of the bladder."

By early 2014, it was time to have my stimulator battery replaced. I was having more pain in my right leg and beginning to have pain in my left leg combined with low back spasms, anxiety, and depression. I was gaining weight and having to use a cane or wheelchair to get around. I had to have a stair lift installed because I was falling on the stairs and there were times I couldn't climb upstairs from the pain in my foot. I was sent for a Functional Capacity Evaluation test to determine if I was able to return to work. I spent the next six days in bed recovering from the extreme pain. I was also having less relief from my stimulator even after multiple reprogramming attempts. X-rays showed that my paddle had shifted, and that surgery would be needed to reposition it. In 2018, I had a stimulator revision that included removal of the paddle, screws, scar tissue, and wires. The prior laminectomy was extended, and a new larger paddle was placed with new wires. I have said that will be the absolute last stimulator related procedure that I will have. It was several weeks before I returned to my normal. By June I was referred to PT again and had been started on a series of lumbar sympathetic blocks.

Late 2018, I spent a week in the hospital with several things going on. I was initially seen in the ER because I couldn't take a deep breath. I was eventually diagnosed with pulmonary edema, reflux, pancreatic horn atrophy, fatty liver, and impaction. Lots of tests later I can no longer take NSAIDs because of the damage to my stomach lining.

I'm caught in a never-ending cycle of doctor appointments, PT, psychology appointments, and relentless pain.

My pain never stops. It has times of less pain and times of more pain, but it's always there. If I have a good day, I overdo it trying to get things done that I put off because of the pain. I have to rest after showering now. After 23-years of marriage, I am divorced. The house in the country we built belongs to someone else. I have to schedule a day to rest before and after going anywhere. I've been yelled at by strangers for parking in handicapped spaces when I go grocery shopping. I've had to ask store associates to bring me an electric cart halfway through shopping when the pain attacked out of nowhere. CRPS has changed every part of my life and it will never get better.

COMPLEX REGIONAL PAIN SYNDROME (CRPS)

AND THE MEDICAL COMMUNITY:

A PATIENT'S PERSPECTIVE

Eric M. Phillips
International RSD Foundation
www.rsdinfo.com

Abstract: Complex regional pain syndrome (CRPS), is a chronic pain disease of the sympathetic nervous system caused by trauma (injury) or surgery that it is poorly understood by the medical community. Many patients may suffer long before getting diagnosed or even receive proper treatment.

From a patient's perspective of suffering from CRPS for over 34-years and helping other CRPS patients for over the past 31-years, it has shown me the difficulties that patients go through in dealing with the medical community.

Many patients, unfortunately, go through being misdiagnosed and provided no treatment for their disease due to the lack of understanding and knowledge of CRPS by the medical community.

Keywords: Complex regional pain syndrome (CRPS), CRPS awareness, CRPS community, and the medical community.

Introduction

Complex regional pain syndrome (CRPS), has been documented in the United States since 1864 during the American Civil War by Doctor Silas Weir Mitchell and as early as the 16th century by Ambroise Paré a French barber surgeon who was one of the first to describe what is now called CRPS, through his account of the persistent pain which King Charles IX had suffered from.

As we know CRPS is not a "new disease." It has been around for over 155-years. Over the years there have been tens of thousands of medical articles that have been written and published on this subject. Also, there have been many name changes to this disease from the first account by Doctor Mitchell when he coined the term Causalgia.

CRPS affects millions of people worldwide. The lack of education and awareness in the medical community can cause the patient many years of much frustration of not being believed, it causes a delay in diagnosis, delay in treatment, and proper care to help control the patient's pain.

There are many ways people can develop CRPS such as, (injury, surgery, venipuncture injury (1), electrical injury, etc.). One has to remember that there are no two cases that are the same.

Most people know this disease by its former name reflex sympathetic dystrophy (RSD). To me, you can call it anything you would like. You can even call it XYZ. It does not matter what name you call it RSD or CRPS, they are the same. One of the most common factors that all CRPS patients share is living in constant chronic pain.

Dealing with the Medical Community

Dealing with the medical community as a CRPS patient can be a challenging aspect of dealing with this disease. This challenge has been difficult for myself and many other CRPS patients worldwide.

Even after the patient receives a proper diagnosis of CRPS, they fall through the cracks because many physicians do not understand the disease or know how to treat such a complex disease.

This causes the patient to see many doctors until they find the right doctor who understands the disease.

Once the patient finds the right doctor, they should be able to receive some form of proper treatment to help with their pain. Some patients may have to see anywhere from 10, 20, or even 30 doctors before they finally find the right doctor who understands and knows how to treat CRPS.

An unfortunate thing that faces many CRPS patients who do not have a treating physician to help manage their chronic pain, is usually forced to visit the Emergency Room (ER) at their local hospital to seek some type of treatment for their pain. The ER is not the best place for patients to seek treatment for their CRPS pain.

The ER is another place where doctors need to be educated on CRPS. Most of the doctors working in the ER have "no clue" of what CRPS is. Their first thoughts are these patients are simply in the ER to seek drugs. This event is not true at all. These patients become so desperate they are forced into visiting the ER to obtain some type of help for their pain because they have no treating physician to manage their care.

Some people in the medical community have made comments that patients are "doctor shopping." These comments are so far from the truth. Unfortunately, patients must go through seeing, so many doctors before they find the right one to receive proper care and help.

As I tell every CRPS patient that I talk to, I mention that they know their body better than anyone in this world. You must find the right doctor who understands this disease and knows how to treat it.

One must find a doctor who has compassion and will treat you like a human. Half the battle of dealing with CRPS is finding a doctor who will understand your disease and treat you with respect. This part of dealing with CRPS goes a long way in my book. The patient must remember they are the ones in charge of their care and treatment. When a patient is with the wrong doctor, they are in for a life of living in more pain, being prescribed unnecessary narcotics, having unnecessary procedures and surgeries.

The Frustrating Part of Dealing with CRPS

The frustrating part of living with CRPS for the past 34-years is when I talk with other patients. They all share similar stories with me that they are not helped or believed by the medical community. This problem is a global epidemic for many in the CRPS community. It does not matter where patients live.

They could live in the United States, Canada, England, France, Australia, New Zealand, The Netherlands or any other country in this world. Patients tell me constantly that their doctors do not believe that CRPS can spread, be that painful, or they think it is all in the patient's head.

I feel the reason these doctors make such statements, is that they are not educated enough on the topic of CRPS. These are some of the reasons why patients are mistreated by the medical community. From the doctor's lack of knowledge, the patients are the ones who suffer most, because they are denied any type of treatment that could be beneficial to help relieve their pain. May it be by performing a nerve block or giving the patient the proper medication to help their pain.

To be honest, there are no so-called "experts" who treat CRPS. I feel that there are a few doctors worldwide I can honestly say have more knowledge than others on the topic of CRPS.

The late Doctor Hooshang Hooshmand (my mentor, teacher, and best friend) once made a statement to me. He said CRPS patients have more knowledge about the disease than most doctors do. This is because the patients are the ones living with the disease. That statement can't be further from the truth.

Nowadays, it is sad to know that there are so many people in the medical community that have no understanding about this complex disease.

Patients and their treating physician must work together to create a treatment plan, which will be beneficial for the patient.

Working as a team to discuss treatment options, can be helpful to the patient in time. The worst thing for the patient is not having a treatment plan.

It is vital that the patient and physician have a good working relationship. The patient needs to have trust and confidence in their treating physician. When there is a treatment plan in place, it makes dealing with such a complex situation much easier for both the patient and physician.

These are the keys to a successful outcome for the patient.

Educating the Medical Community

Education for the medical community must start at the medical college level. One must remember that most medical students are only taught about a chapter (or less) worth of information on CRPS. The medical community must realize that CRPS is a disease that affects millions of patients worldwide. Some doctors say CRPS is a rare disease. It should no longer be considered a rare disease anymore. There are too many cases worldwide for it to be considered a rare disease. It's not like there are only 100 documented cases worldwide. We have millions of people suffering from CRPS worldwide.

Once we have the medical community educated, it will help patients over time, where they can receive proper treatment which can help control their pain and give them some hope.

The other part of educating the medical community is that it can also help promote more research on CRPS. Research is a big key in pursuing a cure for CRPS. It will take many years to decades to research this disease, to help find a complete cure for this unrelenting disease.

Most patients may not see a cure in their lifetime, but one can only hope that with time CRPS can be cured. No one should ever have to live in this much pain.

CRPS Awareness

There needs to be more awareness of CRPS worldwide in both the medical community and the public. Nowadays, you think a disease like CRPS would be a more recognized name worldwide in the medical community, in the public, and the media. CRPS should be a household name by now. It has been documented in the United States for over 155-years. CRPS should have the same recognition as other conditions such as Fibromyalgia, Lyme Disease, Lupus, Multiple Sclerosis, etc...

For example, Fibromyalgia is a household name today, because of the media coverage, and the T.V. Ads it receives from the medication Lyrica. I am puzzled why CRPS does not have the same recognition as other diseases and condition that are household names today?

Many states throughout the United States have a CRPS Awareness Month. Having an awareness month can help give the much-needed recognition to the people who suffer from CRPS.

There needs to be a global CRPS awareness month so that everyone worldwide can gain recognition in areas where patients have no help.

The only way that CRPS can get the same recognition as other conditions such as Fibromyalgia or Lyme's Disease is through awareness. The CRPS community and the medical community must gather with the same goal to help get awareness out there, on how CRPS can affect a person's life.

Conclusion

The most important thing patients need on their side is a medical community that understands every aspect of CRPS. They must understand this disease does spread from limb to limb and other parts of the body (2-10). There are even cases of internal organ involvement. Doctors must learn to understand that a patient does not have to have every sign and symptom of the disease to have it. CRPS affects everyone differently.

As, most patients know their symptoms of CRPS can come and go at any time. It's called the "vicious cycle of pain." This lack of knowledge can harm the patient from getting the proper treatment which can help control their pain.

How would some of these doctors feel if they go into a doctor's office and are told that their health issue is all in their head or it's not real? I am sure they would not like it or even if this disease happened to one of their family members, they would not like it either.

Nowadays, it is sad to know that there are so many people in the medical community that have no understanding about this complex disease.

There are millions of people worldwide suffering daily from the unrelenting pain of CRPS. As we know that there is no magic cure for CRPS now. Maybe, someday, there will be a cure. We need more research into finding a cure for this disease.

This idea will only happen when patients are heard from, and when the doctors take the time to get educated and listen to what the patient is going through with their pain. The main thing is that the medical community has to understand this is a real problem which affects millions of people.

This disease does not discriminate. CRPS can happen to anyone at any time. I have talked to tens of thousands of people over the past 31 plus years. I have heard from doctors, lawyers, ministers, and other professional people who have developed CRPS. No one wants this disease. Heck! If I could change things, I would not want CRPS for the past 34-years either.

Over the past 34-years, I have met many doctors who don't believe in this disease. They make comments like most CRPS patients are only drug seekers, they suffer from some psychological issue or this disease is just a wastebasket diagnosis. These are the comments that give CRPS a bad name.

With the lack of understanding on the doctor's behalf, it places the patient in a difficult position trying to obtain the proper treatment and help.

Many CRPS cases are developed from a work-related injury. When people get hurt on the job, they must deal with workers compensation, and the "not so nice people" at the insurance company. Most patients must go through years of fighting with the insurance companies and the doctors that they are sent to by worker's comp. Patients have to fight tooth and nail for their medications, treatments, and back pay.

This scenario becomes a snowball effect in dealing with doctors and insurance companies that have no understanding of the patient's disease. This type of situation causes the patient more pain and stress trying to deal with doctors and people working at the insurance companies who have no idea what the patient is dealing with. This becomes another downfall for the patient.

The people at the workers compensation and the insurance companies also need to be educated on the topic of CRPS. This fact will make the process much easier for everyone involved.

Patients need to become an advocate in their management of care. There are a few doctors out there that will advocate for their patients, but in most cases, the patient is the sole advocate.

The main goal for every CRPS patient is to be pain-free and to have a better quality of life.

To help solve the problems that CRPS patients face, there needs to be more awareness and education on CRPS. Education and a better understanding are the keys for proper treatment and hope for all CRPS patients.

Doctors should take the time to listen to the "patients' perspective of living in chronic pain." It will help them have a better understanding of what CRPS patients live with daily.

References

1. Hooshmand H, Hashmi M, Phillips EM. Venipuncture complex regional pain syndrome type II. AJPM 2001; 11: 112-124.

2. Hooshmand H, and Phillips EM: Spread of complex regional pain syndrome (CRPS). Source: www.rsdrx.com and www.rsdinfo.com

3. Hooshmand H. Chronic pain: reflex sympathetic dystrophy. Prevention and management. Boca Raton, FL: CRC Press, 1993; pp 1-202.

4. Hooshmand H, and Hashmi H. Complex regional pain syndrome (CRPS, RSDS) diagnosis and therapy. A review of 824 patients. Pain Digest 1999; 9: 1-24.

5. Veldman PH, Goris RJ: Multiple reflex sympathetic dystrophy which patients are at risk for developing a recurrence of reflex sympathetic dystrophy in the same or another limb. Pain 1996; 64:463-466.

6. Schwartzman RJ. Reflex sympathetic dystrophy. Handbook of Clinical Neurology. Spinal Cord Trauma, H.L. Frankel, editor. Elsevier Science Publisher B.V. 1992; 17: 121-136.

7. Schwartzman RJ, McLellan TL: Reflex sympathetic dystrophy. A review. Arch Neurol 1987; 44:555-561.

8. Maleki J, LeBel AA, Bennett GJ, Schwartzman RJ. Patterns of Spread of complex regional pain syndrome, type I (reflex sympathetic dystrophy). Pain 2000; 88: 259-266.

9. Kozin F, McCarty DJ, Sims J, Genant H. The reflex sympathetic dystrophy syndrome. I. Clinical and histologic studies: evidence of bilaterality, response to corticosteroids and articular involvement. Am J Med 1976; 60:321-331.

10. Radt P. Bilateral reflex neurovascular dystrophy following a neurosurgical procedure. Clinical picture and therapeutic problems of the syndrome. Confinia. Neurl 1968; 30 (5): 341-348.

Made in the USA
Middletown, DE
25 January 2020

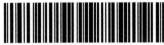

83562525R00132